THE
PESCATARIAN
MEAL PLAN
& COOKBOOK

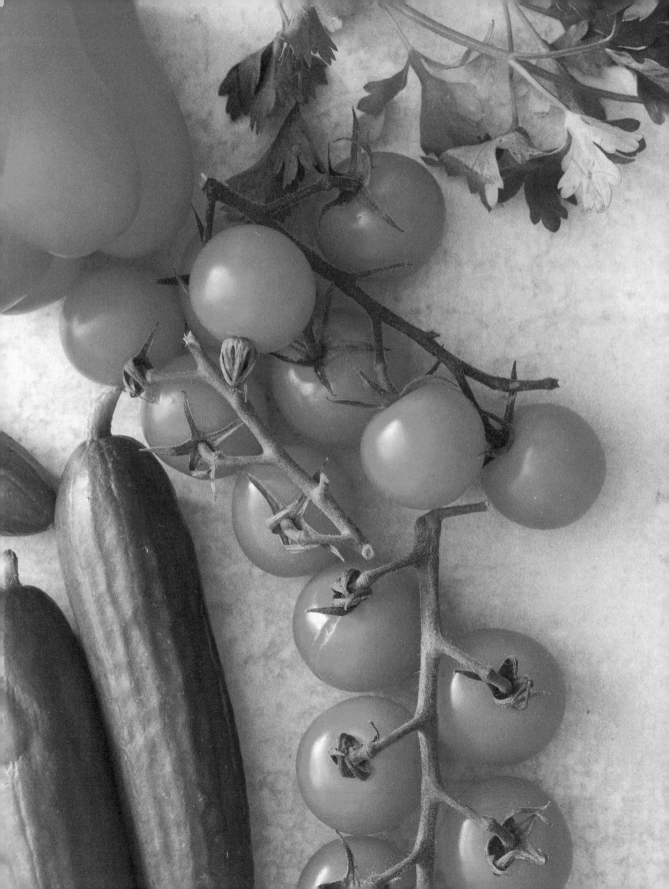

CHELSEY AMER MS, RDN, CDN

PHOTOGRAPHY BY **EVI ABELER**

THE 28-DAY PESCATARIAN MEAL PLAN & COOKBOOK

YOUR GUIDE TO JUMP-STARTING A HEALTHIER LIFESTYLE

ROCKRIDGE
PRESS

For general information on our other products and services or to obtain technical support, please contact our Customer Care Department within the United States at (866) 744-2665, or outside the United States at (510) 253-0500.

Rockridge Press publishes its books in a variety of electronic and print formats. Some content that appears in print may not be available in electronic books, and vice versa.

Interior and Cover Designer: Jay Dea
Art Producer: Janice Ackerman
Editor: Rebecca Markley
Production Editor: Jenna Dutton

Photography: © 2019 Evi Abeler.
Food Styled by Albane Sharrard.
Author Photo: ©2019 Molly Quill

ISBN: Print 978-1-64611-496-2
        eBook 978-1-64611-497-9
R0

To my boys—thank you for your smiles, encouragement, and being my number-one fans. Lex, I hope you find joy, health, and adventure in food, too!

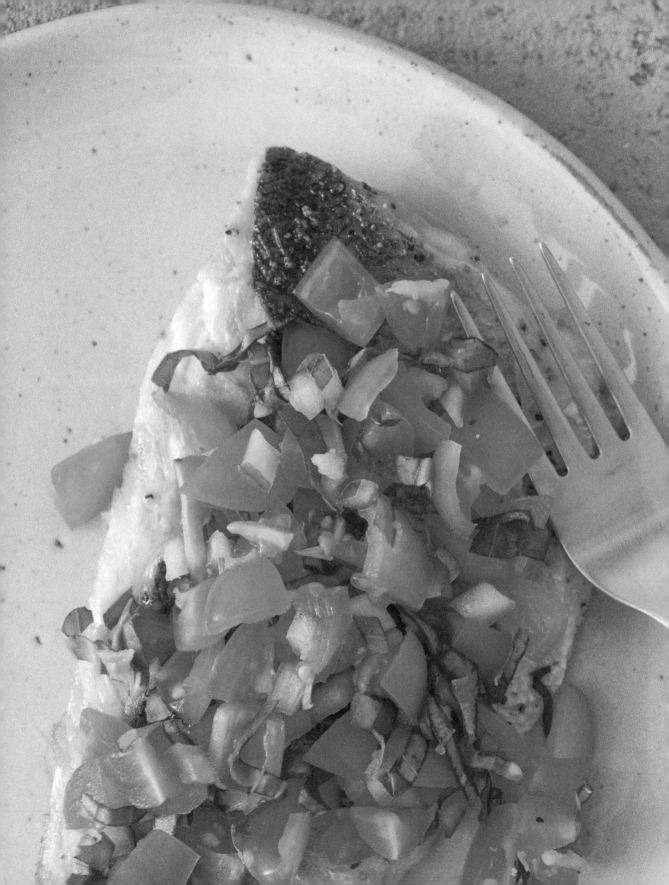

CONTENTS

INTRODUCTION

Are you totally confused about what to eat?

I get it, because I once was, too. There was a time when I ate low carb because I thought it was healthy and would help me lose those stubborn five pounds. Instead, my energy plummeted, my cravings spiked, and I was moody. Then I went vegan because plant-based eating was popular. But a vegan diet didn't work with my food allergies to tree nuts, peanuts, and sesame seeds. Eventually, I started eating eggs and dairy because a restrictive vegan diet wasn't sustainable for me.

When I was in graduate school for nutrition, a lightbulb went off. I didn't have to be overly restrictive to feel good in my body. Adding fish alongside a plant-based diet worked.

We're constantly bombarded with conflicting messages from the media about which diet is best, but in reality, the diet that works for you reigns supreme. As I adopted more of a pescatarian way of eating, my confusion about what to eat vanished. I felt nourished, satisfied, and energized.

Plus, as a registered dietitian, I knew that a pescatarian diet was full of health benefits from reduced risk of chronic diseases, like heart disease and diabetes, to vanity benefits, like strong and shiny skin, hair, and nails, thanks to the abundance of omega-3 fatty acids.

While I strongly believe that there's no one-size-fits-all approach to nutrition, I do believe most people could benefit from eating the pescatarian way.

Why? It's simple, approachable, and doable. Whether you choose to consume mostly plant-based meals with fish sprinkled into your diet or you lean toward a fish-heavy meal plan, the pescatarian diet can work for you. You don't have to spend tons of time in the kitchen or be a master chef to follow the pescatarian lifestyle.

That's why I'm so excited to share this book with you. I wrote and tested these recipes a few months after I had my son and needed to fuel my body properly. I was nursing around the clock, working, and adjusting to life as a new parent. Following the meal plan I created in this book fueled a hectic season of life, without taking much time away from my family.

That's exactly what I hope this book does for you. Most of the recipes can be made in 30 minutes or less with recognizable ingredients you can find in any supermarket. Even more, there's a 28-day meal plan to help you get started. This book isn't just a cookbook. It's a resource to help you adopt the pescatarian diet and make a flexible eating plan work for you.

If you're new to meal planning, the 28-day plan will help you jump-start the pescatarian diet with set meals and snacks, plus shopping lists are included. But there's no pressure to follow the plans to a T to reap the benefits! Customize your meals to your preference or what's convenient for you. By the end of the next month, you will be able to design your own pescatarian menus and meal plans to help fuel *your* current season of life. Let's dive in.

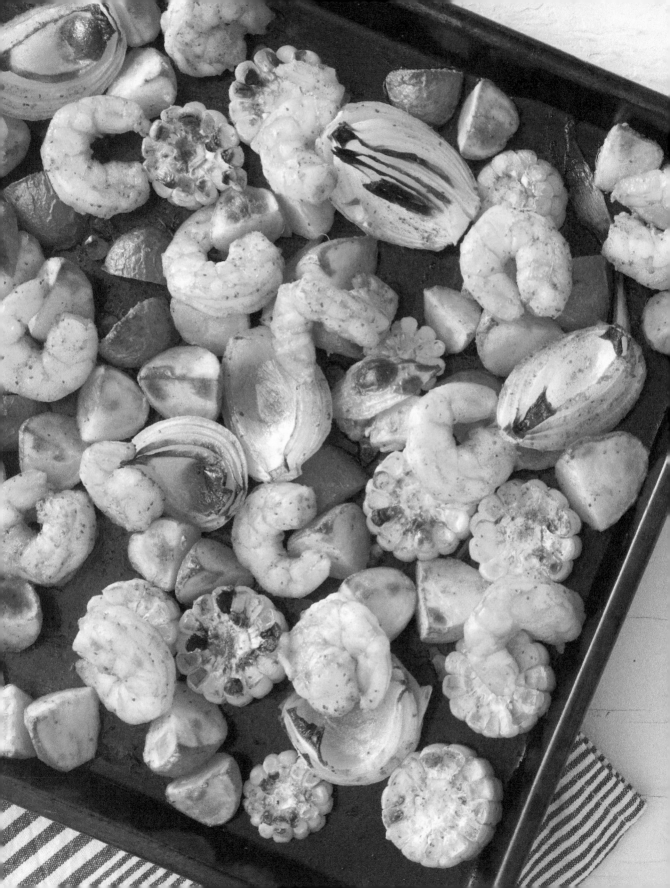

CHAPTER ONE

THE PESCATARIAN DIET

What if there was an eating style that's easy to follow, improves your health, and helps you effortlessly maintain a healthy weight? It almost sounds too good to be true!

But it's not . . . I'm referring to the pescatarian diet.

The term "pescatarian" was introduced in the early 1990s as a hybrid of the Italian word for fish, *pesce*, and "vegetarian." Simply put, a pescatarian diet is a predominantly plant-based pattern of eating, like a vegetarian diet, but it includes seafood as a primary protein source. Pescatarians complete their meals with a variety of vegetables, fruit, legumes, healthy fats, and some whole-grains and dairy. As an inclusive way of eating, pescatarians eat a wide variety of foods, except for red meat and poultry.

Harnessing the proven health advantages of a plant-forward vegetarian diet, with the additional well-studied benefits of the omega-3 fatty acids found in many types of seafood, pescatarians often care about their health and eat the pescatarian way to thrive.

If you want to follow a pescatarian diet, you've come to the right place! Let's explore the pesco-vegetarian way of eating.

THE FIVE GUIDING PRINCIPLES

Instead of a rigid diet with a set plan you must follow, the pescatarian diet is flexible. It's rich in seafood and plant-based proteins and includes a bounty of produce, plus healthy fats and whole-grains. Essentially, it's a whole foods approach to eating. Of course, there's still room for indulgences, too, because the pescatarian way of eating is a lifestyle, not a quick-fix diet plan.

Let's examine the five guiding principles of the pescatarian diet that you should think about as you begin your journey:

1. Choose Seafood at Least Twice Weekly

When selecting your protein source, fish and shellfish should be your primary animal protein. After all, fish ("pesce") is in the name! It is safe for healthy individuals to eat seafood several times weekly. In fact, it's often recommended that you eat *at least* two servings of fish each week. With a wide variety of options and preparations to choose from, it's easy to fill a quarter of your plate with a fish fillet, shrimp, scallops, mussels, and more.

2. Add Plant-Based Proteins to Your Plate

Consider the pescatarian diet primarily a whole foods plant-based way of eating, plus fish. To meet your daily protein needs, incorporate plant-based proteins, including beans, lentils, nuts, seeds, and high-quality soy products like tofu and tempeh, to your weekly meal rotation. Many of these protein sources are low in fat, high in fiber, and packed with vitamins and minerals. Even more, plant-based proteins are often inexpensive and easy to prepare.

3. Eat an Abundance of Vegetables and Fruit

Vegetables and fruit are the cornerstone of a nourishing diet, like the pescatarian diet. By filling your plate with more vegetables and fruit, you'll consume more vitamins and minerals (without popping a pill), plus fiber and water. Enjoy ample vegetables throughout the day, including both raw and cooked produce. No vegetables are off limits, so peruse the aisles of your supermarket or farmer's market and try something new.

4. Focus on Fiber-Filled Carbohydrates

High-fiber diets repeatedly reign supreme to reduce your risk of chronic diseases, including heart disease and diabetes. In addition to vegetables, fruit, beans, and lentils, whole-grains and high-fiber starchy vegetables (potatoes, sweet potatoes, peas, and corn) are superior for your health. Compared to refined grains, whole-grains contain more fiber, B vitamins, iron, magnesium, and even some healthy fats, which all contribute to their health benefits.

5. Include Healthy Fats

On the pescatarian diet, fat is not to be feared. Eating some healthy fats daily promotes better absorption of fat-soluble vitamins, boosts satiety, and contributes to the health-enhancing impact of the pescatarian lifestyle. Choose olive oil, avocado, nuts, and seeds, in addition to fish full of omega-3 fatty acids.

Specifically, the omega-3 fatty acids found in salmon, sardines, herring, halibut, and other fish help lower inflammation. It's been well documented that consuming more omega-3 fatty acids can improve heart health, reduce the risk of a stroke and repeat heart attack, and help control some autoimmune diseases, including lupus and rheumatoid arthritis.

THE HEALTH BENEFITS

Eating the pescatarian way isn't only delicious, but nutritious, too! Studies repeatedly prove that the pescatarian diet leads to superior health outcomes when compared to many other dietary patterns.

Here are just a few of the health advantages you may experience on the pescatarian diet:

Improves Heart Health

Your heart will thank you for eating the pescatarian way! One of the best-studied health benefits of following the pescatarian diet is improved heart health for men and women. Pescatarian diets are rich in omega-3 fatty acids, antioxidants, and fiber, and low in saturated fat. As mentioned above, anti-inflammatory omega-3 fatty acids, coupled with a high intake of vegetables, fruit, and whole-grains contribute to the lower risk of heart disease.

The American Heart Association recommends eating fish twice weekly to reduce your risk of many heart diseases, including coronary heart disease, congestive heart failure, stroke, sudden cardiac death, and more.

Simplifies Weight Management

To lose weight, you must be in a caloric deficit. Eating a plant-rich diet makes this effortless! Many studies have shown that individuals who follow a plant-forward diet, including vegans, vegetarians, and pescatarians, have lower body mass indexes (BMI) compared to their meat-eating counterparts. Why? Likely because pescatarians and vegetarians fill up on more plants, which are low in calories and fat and high in fiber.

Reduces Risk of Type 2 Diabetes

The pescatarian diet is anti-inflammatory, high in omega-3 fatty acids, and rich in fiber, which all contribute to reducing the risk of type 2 diabetes. In fact, in the Adventist Health Study-2 cohort, with more than 70,000 individuals, pescatarians had the greatest flavonoid (a type of antioxidant) intake, which could be why plant-heavy diets may reduce the risk of developing type 2 diabetes by half.

Even more, replacing meat consumption with fish and plant-based proteins proves beneficial for individuals at risk for diabetes. Studies demonstrate an association between red meat consumption and incidence of type 2 diabetes.

Lowers Mortality Rate

A major study found that compared to meat-eaters, pescatarians had significantly lower mortality rates. No wonder the pescatarian lifestyle is growing in popularity! In addition to a plant-powered diet, this may be because of the anti-inflammatory omega-3 fatty acids in fish and a lower saturated fat intake from not eating meat and poultry.

Diminishes Dementia Risk

Eating fish, especially fatty fish rich in omega-3 fatty acids, may benefit your brain health, too. Specifically, consuming fish once weekly was associated with a 60 percent lower risk of Alzheimer's disease, according to a study published in *Archives of Neurology*. This is likely due to boosting your omega-3 fatty acid intake, plus a pescatarian diet is rich in anti-oxidants and low in saturated fat, which may protect against cognitive decline.

Reduces Cancer Risk

Following a vegetarian diet—and, even more precisely, a pesco-vegetarian diet—has been shown to reduce the risk of colorectal cancer (cancers of the colon and rectum). As a leading cause of cancer mortality, it may be especially important for individuals who are at increased risk for colon cancer to follow a pescatarian diet, including men and women over the age of 50, smokers, those with a family history of colon cancer, and individuals of African American or Hispanic descent.

THE SCIENCE BEHIND THE DIET

As you can see, eating the pescatarian way has many benefits, but why is it so healthy?

Put simply, eating a predominantly plant-based diet, plus replacing meat with plant-based proteins and fish, adds beneficial nutrients to your diet. You'll consume more vitamins, minerals, antioxidants, fiber, and omega-3 fatty acids while reducing your intake of saturated fat and added sugars.

Let's examine why this benefits your health.

Antioxidants

A diet rich in antioxidants protects your body against oxidative stress, or the imbalance of free radicals and antioxidants. Free radicals are unstable atoms. Too many free radicals can damage cells and proteins in your body, including your DNA. To simplify matters, the more oxidative stress you have in your body, the greater the likelihood of cellular damage, inflammation, and associated inflammatory diseases, like heart disease, diabetes, cancer, and dementia.

Making vegetables the focus of your meals boosts your intake of vitamins, minerals, and antioxidants. For instance, you'll consume more potassium; magnesium; vitamins A, C, and E; and many more necessary substances. Many individuals don't eat enough of these key nutrients.

Fiber

A diet full of fiber helps protect your body from chronic diseases. A pescatarian diet is rich in whole-grains, vegetables, fruit, and fiber-filled plant-based proteins, like beans, lentils, and legumes. Fiber helps reduce your blood sugar levels, improves your body's insulin response, reduces cholesterol levels, and improves the health and diversity of your gut.

Even more, a high-fiber diet is often associated with lower caloric intake. This can reduce your risk of obesity and make it easier to maintain a healthy weight, which can also improve insulin sensitivity (thus reducing your risk of developing diabetes and heart disease).

Omega-3 Fatty Acids

A cornerstone benefit of the pescatarian diet is high omega-3 fatty acid intake. Eating more fish and less meat and poultry replaces saturated fat consumption with heart-protective omega-3 fatty acids.

There are two main types of omega-3 fatty acids found in fish: EPA (eicosapentaenoic acid) and DHA (docosahexaenoic acid). Many individuals supplement these long-chain omega-3 fatty acids with fish oil supplements, but experts suggest boosting your intake from food.

Countless studies prove the anti-inflammatory benefits of omega-3 fatty acids from fish consumption. Aside from the cardioprotective benefits of boosting your EPA and DHA intake (reduced cholesterol and triglyceride levels, lower risk of cardiac events), sufficient intake may reduce the risk of preterm labor, support muscle recovery, boost eye health, and improve hyperactivity disorders. Even more, there is evidence that omega-3 fatty acids *specifically from fish* may decrease insulin secretion, warding off diabetes.

Saturated Fat and Added Sugars

As a nutrition professional, I prefer to focus on what you add to your diet, but it's important to mention what's limited on a pescatarian diet. Pescatarians consume less saturated fat and added sugars than what's in the typical American diet. Diets high in saturated fat and added sugars are historically linked to chronic inflammatory diseases, like heart disease and diabetes. By replacing your saturated fat and added sugar intake with more beneficial nutrients (like antioxidants, fiber, and omega-3 fatty acids), you'll reap the numerous health benefits mentioned previously.

GOOD FATS VS. BAD FATS

Not all fat is created equally! Two major types of fats found in food are unsaturated fats and saturated fats, which differ based on their chemical structure.

Saturated fat, found in red meat, coconut oil, dairy products, and many packaged and processed foods, is known as the "bad fat" due to its association with increased risk of heart disease and diabetes. Saturated fat is often solid at room temperature.

"Good fats," or *un*saturated fats, structurally contain one or more double bonds. Olive oil, sunflower oil, avocado, olives, nuts and seeds, and fatty fish are predominantly unsaturated fats. Omega-3 fatty acids, a type of unsaturated fat found in fatty fish like salmon, herring, and sardines, have far-reaching benefits in your body to reduce inflammation and inflammatory diseases.

Most individuals don't eat enough omega-3 fatty acids, but experts recommend healthy individuals eat fish at least twice weekly to consume sufficient omega-3 fatty acids.

ADAPTING TO THE PESCATARIAN WAY OF EATING

The best eating plan to help you improve your health is one that you can follow for years. Luckily, it's easy to adopt the pescatarian way of eating.

A picturesque plate on the pescatarian diet may include an abundance of fresh vegetables next to a beautiful piece of fish, paired with a quick-and-easy grain salad. Or perhaps it's a pre-prepped mason jar salad with wild canned salmon. Or maybe it's a plant-based meal of lentil "meatballs" (page 84).

If this doesn't sound like a typical "diet" to you, you're right! The pescatarian diet is not another restrictive fad diet plan that will help you drop weight quickly. It's a *lifestyle* you can adopt and sustain for years that will reduce your risk of chronic diseases like heart disease, diabetes, Alzheimer's disease, certain types of cancer, and more.

The pescatarian diet is doable. It's a way of eating that anyone—yes, that includes you—can follow! You don't need fancy equipment or specialty ingredients. A knife, a sauté pan, and a sheet pan are the basic equipment you need to get started, and you don't need to count calories or macros. Simply choose your meals from an extensive list of ingredients, including vegetables, fruit, seafood, beans, lentils, eggs, whole-grains, healthy fats, and some dairy products. There are endless combinations of tasty meals you can create that will help you reach your health and wellness goals, including more than 60 delicious recipes in this book to help you get started.

Best of all, you don't need to spend excessive time laboring over your food. The pescatarian diet is great to follow if you're short on time in the kitchen or simply don't wish to spend your free time cooking. In fact, 35 recipes in this book can be made in under 30 minutes start to finish! Without struggling over each and every meal, you can easily maintain your weight, improve your health, and enjoy delicious food. You're busy, but you don't need to sacrifice your health because of that!

Foods to Enjoy

As you now know, the pescatarian diet is not a restrictive diet. There is an abundance of foods to enjoy while working towards your health goals. For a long-term lifestyle plan, an assortment of foods is essential to prevent boredom. Plus, a diverse diet means you'll consume a variety of nutrients.

Fill your plate with more of the following:

- Dark leafy greens, such as spinach, kale, and collard greens

- Cruciferous vegetables, including broccoli, cauliflower, and Brussels sprouts

- Starchy vegetables, including potatoes, sweet potatoes, corn, winter squashes, and peas

- Berries, such as blueberries, raspberries, strawberries, and blackberries

- Fatty fish, such as salmon, halibut, tuna, mackerel, and sardines

- Shellfish, including shrimp, scallops, crab, mussels, clams, and lobster

- Plant-based proteins, including beans, lentils, nuts, and seeds

- Whole-grains, such as farro, oats, and quinoa

- Healthy fats, including olive oil, avocado, olives, nuts, and seeds

Foods to Limit

The pescatarian lifestyle is one of inclusion; however, there are certain foods to limit. By definition, the pescatarian diet avoids red meat, poultry, and wild game. By avoiding these animal products, the pescatarian diet is lower in saturated fat compared to carnivorous diets. Choose fish, shellfish, and plant-based proteins to replace these animal proteins.

In order to reap the health benefits of the pescatarian diet, limit your intake of added sugar. Eating too much added sugar can have negative consequences for your health. You'll increase your risk of obesity, diabetes, heart disease, and more. While some added sugar is completely okay to consume (and included in some recipes throughout this book), it's important to avoid an excessive intake of added sugars. In the United States, added sugars are most often found in sugar-sweetened beverages, desserts, premade sauces and marinades, and processed and packaged foods.

Building the Pescatarian Plate (Portions)

Now that you're well-versed in how the pescatarian diet can benefit your health, let's discuss how to translate the pescatarian diet to your plate. As previously mentioned, there's no need to count calories or excessively use measuring utensils when following the pescatarian way of eating. Instead, you just need a plate!

To start, divide your plate in half. Fill half of your plate with vegetables (or fruit at breakfast). By filling half of your plate with veggies, you'll automatically create a plant-heavy meal to reap the pescatarian lifestyle benefits. Choose raw or cooked vegetables, like the Shaved Fennel, Corn, and Peach Salad (page 60), 10-Vegetable Soup (page 72), or one of the veggie sides in chapter 8 (page 131).

Divide the remaining half of your plate in half again. Fill one-quarter of your plate with protein. Most healthy individuals need about three to six ounces of protein at each meal. As you know, the pescatarian diet includes fish and seafood along with plant-based proteins, such as beans, tofu, lentils, nuts, and seeds. To estimate your protein portions, choose a fish fillet that's about the length of your hand, tofu the size of a deck of cards, or one-half cup beans or lentils (about half of a tennis ball).

The final quarter of your plate should consist of a starchy carbohydrate, such as grains, potatoes, sweet potatoes, corn, peas, or beans. To reap the benefits of the pescatarian diet, choose a starchy carbohydrate that is high in fiber. More often than not, opt for whole-grains over refined white grains.

Common Questions and Concerns for Newcomers (FAQs)

1. Fish can be high in mercury and other heavy metals. Should I be concerned about mercury intake on the pescatarian diet?

For most healthy individuals, it is safe and beneficial to consume fish several times each week. Choose a variety of fish and shellfish to reap the numerous health benefits. Be cautious of the seven fish species highest in mercury: shark, swordfish, bigeye tuna, king mackerel, tilefish, marlin, and orange roughy. It is recommended to limit consumption of these species and avoid completely if you are pregnant or breastfeeding.

The Food and Drug Administration (FDA) and the Environmental Protection Agency (EPA) issue guidance for safe seafood consumption for at-risk individuals, including pregnant and breastfeeding women and young children due to concerns over mercury ingestion. They recommend pregnant and breastfeeding women consume 8 to 12 ounces of a variety of fish low in mercury each week to consume sufficient omega-3 fatty acids and protein. Some of the best choices include salmon, haddock, black sea bass, shrimp, scallops, whitefish, oysters, crab, and cod. For a complete list of the best choices and fish to avoid, visit FDA.gov/media/102331/download.

2. How do I make the most sustainable seafood choices?

Due to destructive fishing practices, some fish species are in danger. However, you can make sustainable seafood choices that benefit you and the environment. There are several resources available to help you make the most sustainable seafood selections, including The Monterey Bay Aquarium Seafood Watch and the NOAA Fish Watch. Both resources contain "Best Choices" lists, as well as "Good Alternatives" and "Avoid" lists so you can be an educated consumer.

When shopping, speak with your fishmonger about the origin of the fish you're purchasing and/or look for sustainable seafood certifications. The following logos suggest that the product is sustainably and responsibly caught/farmed:

- Aquaculture Stewardship Council (ASC) (for farmed fish)
- Marine Stewardship Council (MSC) (for wild-caught fish)
- Best Aquaculture Practices (BAP) (for farmed fish)
- Alaska Seafood Certified Responsible Fisheries (for wild-caught fish)
- Fair Trade USA

3. What's the difference between wild-caught and farm-raised seafood?

Simply put, wild-caught seafood is caught from a lake, ocean, river, the fish's natural habitat. Farm-raised seafood is raised in a tank on a fish farm (referred to as "aquaculture").

Although wild-caught fish is often referred to as "good" and farm-raised fish as "bad," it's not that clear cut. There are many fish farms with sustainable aquaculture practices that make seafood in the United States affordable and available.

Nutritionally, wild-caught fish is often lower in fat and calories because they eat a natural diet. However, farmed fish can be higher in omega-3 fatty acids, if fed a fortified feed.

4. Do I need a supplement on the pescatarian diet?

A pescatarian diet is a well-balanced and diverse diet. For most healthy individuals following a pescatarian diet, a vitamin and mineral supplement is not needed; however, always consult with your healthcare professional.

5. Is canned fish safe for consumption?

Yes! Canned fish is an excellent budget-friendly way to include seafood in your diet. Canned fish is processed and safely sealed (typically with heat) in a can. Although not as fresh as a fillet you may purchase at your supermarket, canned fish is nutritious, affordable, convenient, and easy to prepare for quick meals.

Eating canned fish can be a great way to meet your protein and omega-3 fatty acid needs. In fact, canned fish goes way beyond tuna. Try canned sardines for a dose of vitamin D and vitamin B_{12}, wild canned salmon for a more affordable way to choose wild fish, or canned clams for their iron and potassium content.

6. What are the most budget-friendly fish options?

Cost shouldn't be an obstacle for you to be a successfully practicing pescatarian. There are budget-friendly ways for you to participate in the pescatarian lifestyle:

- Pick plant-based proteins. Eat fish a couple of times weekly, but then also include a variety of plant-based proteins, like beans, lentils, tofu, or tempeh, many of which can be found in the dishes in chapter 6, along with eggs and dairy.

- Rely on canned fish and seafood.

- Choose frozen over fresh. It's often less expensive, but just as nutritious.

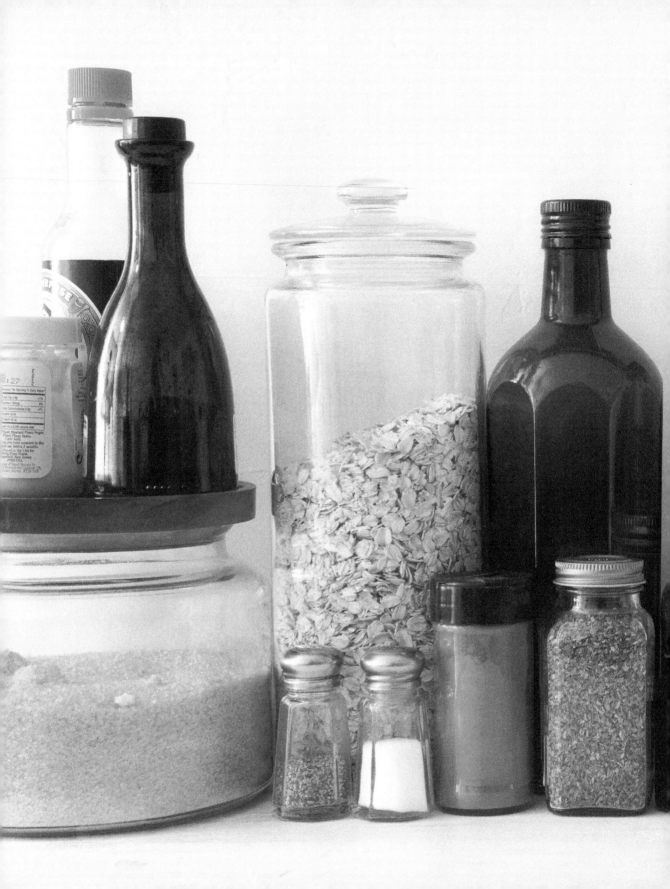

CHAPTER TWO

PREPARING YOUR PESCATARIAN KITCHEN

As a dietitian, one of my favorite catchphrases is "Proper planning provides for peak performance!" While it may be hard to say that five times fast, it couldn't be truer than when developing healthy eating habits, like adopting the pescatarian diet.

Without preparation, it's easy to make excuses. Think about it—how many times have you said something like "I don't have beans [or insert any pantry item], so I can't make the bean tacos [or any recipe] I planned. I'll just order takeout instead." One missed dinner turns into two, which turns into several. You forget to restock your pantry, and over time you begin to feel the effects of too much takeout. You're lethargic, bloated from excess salt, and even pack on a few unwanted pounds.

Instead, be prepared for success on the pescatarian diet: stock your pantry, take inventory, and get organized. This way, you'll feel confident in what you're doing. Having a well-stocked kitchen and pantry helps eliminate common obstacles and improves your organization. Frequently used ingredients will be available, you'll cut trips to the super-market in half, and you'll save time and money. Even more, studies show that being organized can help improve your healthy eating habits and boost your energy, so let's get started.

STOCKING THE ESSENTIALS

Setting a good foundation in your kitchen will help spur your success in adopting the pescatarian lifestyle. First, get prepared. Read this chapter to learn about the essentials for optimal success. Second, take inventory of your current pantry, refrigerator, and freezer. You may have more than you think! Surveying your inventory will help you save money by avoiding duplicate purchases. This is also a good time to toss expired pantry items (or those with too much freezer burn). Organize your pantry using the "first in, first out" system to prevent waste in the future. Place items with a sooner expiration date closer to the front and those with a later date behind them. Next, eliminate what you don't need or use. Donate these items to a local food pantry. Finally, stock up to save time later. Head to the store to restock your pantry, refrigerator, and freezer with the necessities to succeed on a pescatarian plan.

The Pantry

Canned beans: Canned beans are one of the most flexible and inexpensive plant-based proteins to stock in your pantry. Full of fiber, too, canned beans can be used in salads, soups, snacks, main dishes, and even desserts (you must try the Blender Black Bean Brownies on page 157).

Canned salmon: As an inexpensive alternative to fresh-caught salmon, canned salmon is packed with protein, omega-3 fatty acids, and even calcium (if it contains bones). For a fraction of the price, you can always eat the pescatarian way if you have canned salmon (and other fish, like sardines and tuna) in your pantry.

Chia seeds: These tiny black seeds are a nutritious superstar and versatile in the kitchen. Sprinkle them on any dish for an extra nutritious boost as they contain a balance of healthy fats, plant-based protein, and fiber. Plus, when added to liquid, chia seeds gel, absorbing up to nine times their weight in liquid and creating a pudding-like texture.

Diced canned tomatoes: Did you know that US-grown canned tomatoes go from farm to can within hours? This locks in their nutrients, including lycopene, vitamins C and E, and potassium, so you get the most out of this seasonal fruit. Plus, canned tomatoes contain more of the antioxidant lycopene than fresh tomatoes, which helps reduce inflammation and ward off chronic diseases.

Dry whole-grains (farro, buckwheat, bulgur, quinoa, etc.): Whole-grains are a staple on the pescatarian diet because they're high in fiber, vitamins, and minerals. Replacing refined white grains with whole-grains will boost your heart health, improve blood sugar control, and more. There are more than 20 types of whole-grains to choose from, so have fun experimenting over time.

Quality oils: Not all oils are created equally. Opt for pure heart-healthy oils rich in mono-unsaturated fats, like olive oil and avocado oil. Avocado oil is the preferred option for higher cooking temperatures because of its higher smoke point, while olive oil is used in dressings and marinades; however, both can safely be used interchangeably.

Rolled oats: A deliciously nutritious breakfast staple, multipurpose oats are rich in fiber, B vitamins, magnesium, iron, and more, plus they're inexpensive.

Spices: A well-stocked spice rack is one of the easiest ways to enhance the flavor of your meal without adding fat or calories. Many spices contain unique health benefits from warding off the common cold to easing digestive discomfort. If you're just building your spice cabinet, start with the basics—salt, pepper, garlic powder, oregano, cinnamon, red pepper flakes, smoked paprika, cumin, chili powder, and curry powder.

The Refrigerator

Avocados: Rich in healthy fats, fiber, and antioxidants, avocados are a "superfood" you should have on hand to mash on toast, add to smoothies, turn into sauces and dressings, throw in a salad, or use in burgers like the Tuna Avocado Burgers (page 122). When shopping find, avocados that are soft to squeeze, but not mushy. If you remove the stem at the top, it should be green, not brown.

Eggs: Eggs are a quick, easy, and versatile protein source to stock in your refrigerator. When possible, look for the terms "organic," "free-range," and "no added hormones." Although "pasture-raised" is not a regulated term, these eggs have been found to contain more anti-inflammatory omega-3 fatty acids and vitamin D.

Fresh fish and shellfish: You'll learn how to select the best fish later in the chapter, but always ask your fishmonger what's freshest when at the fish counter.

Fresh herbs: Add fresh herbs for a bright burst of flavor and plenty of health benefits, too. Parsley, cilantro, dill, rosemary, and thyme are just a few favorites featured throughout the recipes in this book.

Fruit: Most Americans do not consume the recommended two to three servings of fruit per day. Stock your refrigerator with your favorites so you always have an easy snack option. Berries, apples, and pears contain the most fiber, but also shop for melons, bananas, and stone fruits for variety.

Organic tofu: Tofu is an excellent source of plant-based protein and calcium, which is why it's perfect for the pescatarian diet. Organic tofu is inexpensive and GMO-free.

Vegetables: You can't go wrong when stocking your refrigerator with vegetables. When shopping, your cart should look like a rainbow.

The Freezer

Frozen fish: Frozen fish is an affordable way to incorporate seafood into your diet. Minimal nutrients, if any, are lost in the freezing process.

Frozen fruit: Frozen fruit is typically more affordable than fresh, and it's a great option for off-season fruit. It's picked and frozen at its peak ripeness, which also means its peak nutrient content.

Frozen vegetables: If you often let fresh vegetables spoil, opt for frozen! Picked, processed, and frozen at their peak ripeness, frozen vegetables are an excellent alternative to fresh.

The Hardware

You don't need a Michelin-star-worthy kitchen to follow the pescatarian diet. Aside from an oven and stove, plus basic kitchen utensils (like a spatula, ladle, and tongs), here are five kitchen essentials that will help you eat the pescatarian way:

Nesting mixing bowls: Whether you're making a salad, mixing cookie dough, or prepping vegetables to roast, a set of nesting mixing bowls will be helpful in your kitchen. If possible, find a set with matching lids for easy storage in your refrigerator.

Parchment paper: For easy cleanup, parchment paper is a must-have in your pescatarian kitchen. Line sheet pans with parchment paper when roasting vegetables or baking fish to reduce cleaning time. Preparing fish *en papillote*, or in a pouch made from parchment paper, is a simple and quick technique, too.

Sauté pan or cast iron pan: The best way to get crispy skin on fish is to pan-sear it on your stovetop. A heavy sauté pan or cast iron pan is the best kitchen tool to use for this. Bonus points if your pan is oven safe!

Sharp chef's knife: Investing in a good chef's knife, and knowing how to use it, will make prep time a breeze! Alongside a good knife, having a sturdy cutting board that doesn't slide with each cut is important.

Sheet pans: Whether you're roasting, baking, or broiling, sheet pans are necessary to get the job done. Look for rimmed sheet pans to prevent spills in your oven.

SMART SPENDING

The pescatarian diet can cost a pretty penny since seafood is one of the most expensive proteins available. You can be a smart shopper and spend less, however, by following these tips:

1. **Plan your meals to avoid waste.** By following the meal plans in chapter 3 or making your own, you'll prevent food waste and buy only what you need and will use for the week.

2. **Choose frozen over fresh.** Frozen seafood, vegetables, fruit, and even grains can be more affordable than their fresh counterparts. In fact, much of the fish you see "fresh" at the fish counter was previously frozen (check the signs and ask your fishmonger). Even more, you don't have to worry about waste as much when buying frozen foods, since they last longer and don't have to be used right away.

3. **Eat seasonally.** In-season produce and fish are less expensive, so plan your meals accordingly. For example, in many parts of the country crab season is in the fall and winter. Reserve your crab intake for these months to get the biggest bang for your buck!

4. **Use a bulk frozen fish delivery service.** There are several frozen food delivery services that allow you to purchase high-quality fish and shellfish in bulk at discounted prices. As previously discussed, frozen is just as nutritious as fresh, so don't be shy about using these services (if you have the freezer space).

5. **Shop for staples online.** Oftentimes, buying nonperishable staples, including dry grains, canned beans, canned tomatoes, canned fish, and oil online can save you money. Just as you may price-compare your local supermarkets, shop around online between different vendors to find the best deals.

SELECTING AND PREPARING FISH AND SEAFOOD

Is preparing fish and shellfish intimidating to you? You're not alone.

Maybe it's the scaly skin, hard shells, or googly eyes staring back at you. Perhaps it's fear of a fishy scent lingering throughout your home. Or maybe previous attempts resulted in a dry, overpriced home experiment that didn't turn out favorably. Whatever fishy beliefs you may have, purchasing, preparing, and cooking seafood is much easier than you think.

In fact, you don't have to worry about many of these common obstacles if you're just getting started. There are foolproof ways to master cooking fish at home.

First, choose a doable recipe. Instead of attempting to cook a whole fish, try baking a flaky fish fillet, like the Slow-Roasted Dijon Arctic Char (page 104). In place of preparing mussels or clams, choose an easier shellfish, like peeled and deveined shrimp, to boost your confidence. Get help at the fish counter. You don't need to fillet and debone your own fish to be successful. Second, choose an affordable option to ease your fears of wasting money. Start with frozen or canned seafood to get your feet wet. Last, be sure to stay focused in the kitchen. Fish has a short cooking time, which makes it easy to go from flaky fillet to dry and overcooked quickly, but there's no need to be intimidated. Don't leave the kitchen while your fish cooks and avoid multitasking. As a guide, your fish is fully cooked when it becomes opaque and the flesh flakes when pressed with a fork.

And remember, if at first you don't succeed, try and try again. There are so many fish varieties available, the fish counter is your oyster (pun intended)!

Selecting Fish and Seafood

There are many options available when choosing fish and seafood. Do you want to prepare a whole fish or individual fillets? Are you willing to clean, devein, and deshell shellfish? Plus, how can you best determine if the fish is fresh at your market?

One of the best ways to be sure you're purchasing the freshest fish is to befriend your fishmonger. Individuals behind the fish counter are most familiar with your options available and would love to explain the differences between species, preparation suggestions, and freshness of the fish. It's absolutely acceptable to ask when the fish arrived in the store, as freshness of fish quickly declines once caught.

FRESH FISH

Preparing fish fillets is usually easier than a whole fish, especially if you're new to cooking seafood. A benefit of fillets is that your fish purveyor will clean, descale, and debone the fish for you, so all you need to do is choose how to cook it.

When buying whole fish or fillets, pay attention to the following characteristics of fresh fish:

Smell: The freshest seafood shouldn't smell fishy! It should smell fresh. Yes, it may smell like the ocean, but the scent shouldn't be offensive.

Scales and skin: When fish has scales or skin still on, look for tight scales that are close together. The skin should be shiny, not dull.

Eyes: If choosing a whole fish, be sure to check the eyes. Fresh fish should have bright, clear, bulging eyes. If the eyes appear dull or sunken in, pass on it.

Flesh: When buying a fillet, check the flesh. It should be firm and bounce back. Avoid any fillets where an indentation remains when you press into it.

Color: The flesh of your fish should have even coloring throughout. A pink fish, like salmon or arctic char, should be pink throughout with no white patches. White fish, like cod and snapper, should be white, without darkened areas.

PREVIOUSLY FROZEN FISH

It must be listed if the fish was previously frozen. Frozen fish is a great option, and usually more affordable, but "previously frozen" fish typically needs to be cooked quickly once purchased. A never-before-frozen fresh fillet can be frozen if you don't get a chance to use it ASAP.

SHELLFISH

When purchasing shrimp, crab, or lobster, it is usually easiest to buy it with the shell off, as it likely be cleaned and ready to cook, cutting down on your preparation time. Shrimp must also be deveined, so if you're unfamiliar with how to do this, be sure to choose deveined, shell-off options. Some other considerations when buying shellfish include:

Count: When purchasing shrimp, the "count" refers to the number of shrimp per pound. Therefore, the smaller the count means the larger the shrimp size. For example, if buying 16/20 shrimp, you can expect 16 to 20 shrimp per pound. Alternatively, if purchasing 31/40 shrimp, there will be 31 to 40 smaller shrimp per pound.

Open or closed shell: When buying mussels and clams, the shells should be tightly closed. After you bring mussels or clams home from the market, go through your selection before cooking and discard any open shells.

FISH FLAVORS

FISH/SEAFOOD	FLAVOR PROFILES	FLAVORS/SPICES THAT PAIR BEST
Salmon or Arctic char	Buttery texture and flavor because of high fat content. Arctic char is fishier than salmon.	Mustard, smoky flavors, garlic, brown sugar rub, East Asian flavors
White fish (e.g., tilapia, flounder, snapper, cod, bass, grouper, halibut)	Mild fish flavor. Great option for new fish eaters.	Lemon, butter, garlic, Mediterranean flavors (oregano, parsley, capers, olives), basil pesto, Cajun spices, jerk seasoning
Shrimp and lobster	Mildly sweet flavor, tender	East Asian flavors, like soy sauce; smoky flavors, including barbecue sauce or smoked paprika; butter sauces; curry
Mussels and clams	Flavored like the sea, a bit salty and briny	Best prepared in soups and stews
Crab	Sweet, slightly like the ocean	Old Bay Seasoning, Mediterranean flavors, citrus, butter
Tuna	Fishy	East Asian flavors, like soy sauce; garlic; citrus

Preparing Fish and Seafood

Preparing seafood is much simpler than you may think. Here are some top tips to consider:

Buy the freshest fish available. Use the previous tips to ensure your fish is as fresh as possible.

Store fish safely and use it quickly. After returning from the supermarket, immediately store fish in the refrigerator, preferably on the bottom shelf. It is best to use within a day or two of purchase, as the quality of fish declines rapidly after it's caught.

Defrost frozen fish properly. For optimal results, leave plenty of time (about 24 hours) for fish to defrost. Ideally, thaw fish in a bowl in the refrigerator overnight. For a quick thaw, place fish in a plastic bag and submerge in a bowl of cold water or place under cold running water.

Pat fish dry before adding to your pan. For best results when pan-searing fish, be sure your fish is dry. Using paper towels is the easiest and safest way to do this.

Season fish properly. Before cooking, always season fish with salt and pepper, plus additional desired spices or sauces.

Do not marinate fish. Except for tough fish, like a tuna steak, it is best to avoid marinating fish. Delicate varieties will not hold up well in a marinade. Most marinades have acid, which cooks fish, like a ceviche. Unless you're purposely making ceviche, avoid marinating fish and rely on adding sauces and spices just before or during the cooking process.

Babysit your fish once cooking begins. Fish cooks quickly. To avoid an overcooked and rubbery result, watch your fish carefully while cooking. Generally, cook fish on the stovetop for about 10 minutes per inch of thickness. When baking or broiling fish, it may be longer.

Cooking Your Fish and Seafood

Cooking fish and seafood takes mere minutes, which is why it's an easy weeknight staple. Plus, there are countless ways to cook seafood, including the following:

Oven roasting, baking, or broiling: This is one of the easiest ways to prepare fish. Preheat the oven, season your fish, and roast, bake, or broil. What's the difference between roasting and baking? Roasting is at temperatures above 375°F and baking is below. Most fish cooks in the oven for about 15 to 20 minutes. Switch the oven to broil to get a crispy exterior.

Cooking en papillote: One of my favorite ways to recommend beginners cook fish is *en papillote*, or in a pouch, because it's hard to mess up. Wrap fish and veggies in a parchment paper packet to bake. The fish and veggies will steam within the packet. Bake for about 15 to 20 minutes, depending on the thickness of the fish.

Grilling: Firing up the grill is the ultimate summer treat. For best results, choose a sturdy fish with a thicker skin, like salmon, halibut, or tuna. Be sure to oil the grill grates to prevent sticking. For a fun grilling twist, make seafood kebabs using scallops or shrimp. You can also grill a whole fish.

Pan-searing: Use a heavy pan, like a cast iron skillet, for best results. Be sure to preheat the pan before adding the fish to create a crispy exterior. Always begin cooking fish skin-side down. Allow fish to cook three-quarters of the way through skin-side down before carefully flipping to finish on the flesh side.

Steaming: Steaming fish is a quick preparation method that doesn't have to be bland. Fill a pot with one inch of water, then add the seasoned fish to a steaming basket over it. Steam fish for just five to eight minutes, until flaky. Steamed shrimp are ideal for salads and snacks, like a shrimp cocktail. Lobster is also often steamed (about seven minutes per pound).

Poaching: Poached fish is optimal for a tender result. Poaching is a method of cooking fish submerged in simmering liquid. You can use water, but also broth, fish stock, tomato soup, wine, or even oil. Flaky white fish and fattier fish both poach well.

Preparing a whole fish: Once you master cooking a fillet, try roasting a whole fish. At the fish counter, ask for the fish to be prepared for oven-roasting whole, which includes scaling, gutting, and rinsing the fish. All you'll have to do at home is season the exterior with salt and pepper, then stuff the fish with herbs, spices, and aromatics (like lemon, parsley, and garlic). Roast in a 450°F oven for 15 to 20 minutes, depending on the size of the fish, or grill over medium heat for 10 minutes on each side.

Storing Your Fish and Seafood

There's a lot of confusion about safe handling and storage of fish. Here are a few rules of thumb to follow for safety, freshness, and ideal taste:

- Cook fish within one or two days of purchase. If you do not cook within that time, freeze the fish (if not previously frozen). Raw frozen fish can last two to six months in the freezer, depending on the variety.

- You can freeze cooked fish by wrapping it in parchment paper and freezing it in a plastic freezer storage bag. Fish will keep frozen for about one month; however, texture will not be as tender and flaky as when eaten fresh. For best results, reheat in the oven, wrapped in aluminum foil or parchment paper with a few tablespoons of liquid.

- Fish is best eaten when prepared, but you can store leftovers in the refrigerator for up to three days.

- Vacuum-packed smoked salmon in plastic can keep in your refrigerator for up to two months. Once opened, you have about three days to consume.

COOKING TIME AND PORTION QUICK REFERENCE

FISH/ SEAFOOD	THICKNESS, OUNCES PER PORTION, ETC.	OVEN ROASTING, BAKING, OR BROILING	GRILLING	PAN-SEARING OR SAUTÉING	STEAMING	POACHING	WHOLE FISH
SALMON	4 to 6 ounces per portion; 1½- to 2-inches thick	15 to 20 minutes	15 minutes	15 minutes	5 to 6 minutes	15 minutes	Varies
WHITE FISH (i.e., tilapia, flounder, snapper, cod, bass, grouper, halibut)	4 to 6 ounces; ¾-inch thick	10 minutes	8 to 10 minutes	7 to 9 minutes	10 minutes	10 minutes	20 minutes at 450°F
SHRIMP	4 to 6 ounces, 5 to 6 shrimp for 2½₅ count per pound; 8 to 9 shrimp for 3⅓₅ count per pound	Broil for 6 to 7 minutes, until opaque	2 to 3 minutes on each side	2 to 3 minutes on each side	2 to 5 minutes	3 to 5 minutes	N/A
CRAB	4 to 6 ounces crab meat	25 minutes (for legs)	25 to 30 minutes on indirect heat	10 minutes	20 to 30 minutes	5 to 6 minutes for legs	15 minutes
MUSSELS and CLAMS	1 pound per person	N/A	6 to 8 minutes on grill rack, until shells open	Sauté for 5 to 7 minutes, until shells open	5 to 10 minutes, until shells open	5 to 10 minutes, until shells open	N/A

Fish to Skip

There are several species of fish it is best to avoid due to heavy-metal toxicity, over-fishing, and sustainability.

Shark: Sharks absorb heavy metals through their skin and diet. Big fish typically eat smaller fish. Over time, the mercury level in sharks becomes astronomical. For safety, it is best to avoid this fish, especially when pregnant or breastfeeding.

Eel: Typically found on sushi menus (sometimes labeled "unagi"), eel is a species to avoid, according to the Monterey Bay Aquarium's sushi guide. Not only is eel overfished, but it also contains contaminants like PCBs (polychlorinated biphenyls, a man-made chemical), which can disrupt proper hormonal balance in humans.

Swordfish: Like shark, swordfish contains elevated mercury levels and is best to avoid, especially when pregnant or breastfeeding. For similar reasons, it is also recommended to avoid bigeye tuna, king mackerel, tilefish, marlin, and orange roughy when pregnant or nursing.

Farmed and imported catfish: Known to be raised in poor farming conditions, be wary of imported catfish. In the past several years, European countries and the United States have turned away tens of thousands of pounds of catfish due to drug contamination, which contributes to antibiotic resistance.

Chilean seabass: Due to overfishing and elevated mercury levels, Chilean seabass should be avoided. It is considered an endangered species, too.

Unknown local-caught fish (by family and friends): It is best to avoid the unknown when it comes to fish and seafood to avoid unnecessary heavy-metal exposure, potential contaminants, and overfished species.

To learn more about sustainable fishing practices, visit the Seafood Watch Consumer Guides: SeafoodWatch.org/seafood-recommendations/consumer-guides.

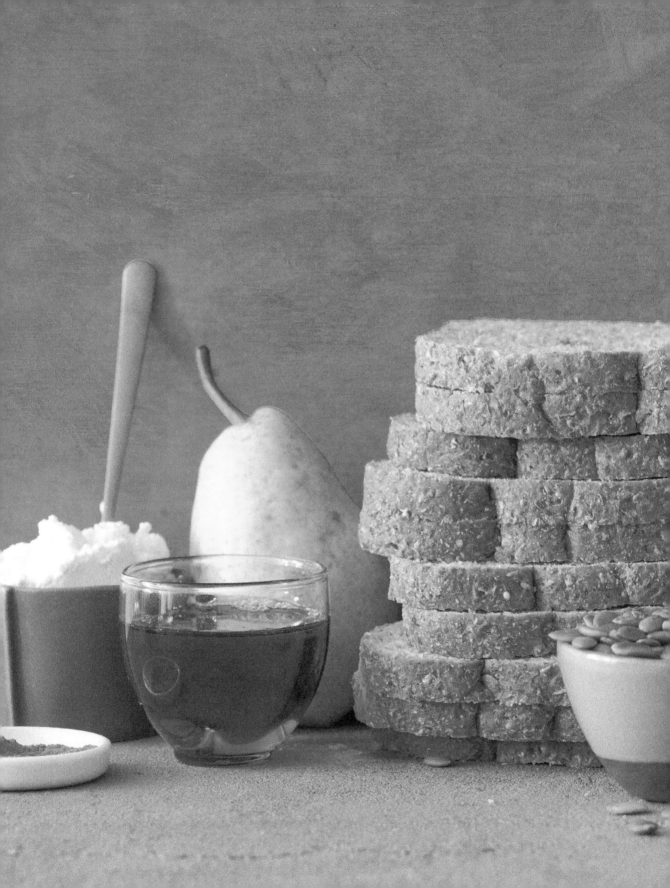

CHAPTER THREE

THE 28-DAY PESCATARIAN MEAL PLAN

Planning is key to success. You wouldn't walk into a boardroom without preparing for a presentation, would you? Treat your health the same way.

When adopting new eating habits, planning is crucial. You may not be able to successfully "wing it" at first—that's okay and expected. Anything that's worth doing—like improving your health—has a learning curve.

Not all planning looks the same, however. For some, planning may be writing a quick dinner plan. For others, it may be a detailed shopping list. Even more, for some it may be actual prep time in the kitchen or making specific recipes before a hectic week begins.

Here are some ways to make meal planning and prep work for you, no matter which type of prep works for you and your family:

1. Set realistic expectations. If you've never spent time planning and preparing your meals before, it's unrealistic for you to plan 21 meals plus snacks for the week. Instead, focus on one meal per day. For example, start with dinner. Choose two to three dinner recipes from this book and enjoy leftovers on the other evenings. You may need to "bulk up" your leftovers with a fresh side or salad, so plan for that, too. Once you master one meal per day, you can add in others. There are a couple of make-ahead breakfast recipes in chapter 4 that are great additions to your weekly prep.

2. Make a shopping list. How many times have you returned home from shopping to realize you forgot the [insert any food here]? It's too easy to forget something without a list. Spend 10 minutes each week to take inventory of your pantry, then write down what you need. Even better, you can keep a running list on your phone of the pantry essentials (see pages 33–34) you need as you run out. When you go to the store with a list, you tend to make healthier choices and spend less (fewer impulse purchases). Plus, you'll waste less food and make quicker trips.

3. Consider shopping online. Online food shopping is one of the best inventions since sliced bread! You can't get distracted by shiny new products or indulgences. You add your items to your cart, select your delivery time, and get cooking when your groceries arrive at your door.

4. Check the weekly sales. Seafood can be expensive, so before planning the week, check local circulars or online sales to minimize costs and make an affordable meal plan.

5. Have a plan in the kitchen. If you choose to set aside a chunk of time to meal prep for the week, enter the kitchen with a plan. I suggest starting with the item that takes the most time to cook.

6. Plan for deviations. Life happens—soccer practice may run late or you may not want what's planned one evening. Having go-to backup options, such as any of the recipes labeled "30 Minutes," will help you successfully deviate from your plan.

THE FIRST WEEK

DAY	BREAKFAST	LUNCH	DINNER
1	Zucchini Bread Baked Oatmeal (page 50)	Easy Israeli Shrimp Salad (page 61)	Sheet Pan Miso Honey Tempeh and Broccoli (page 86)
2	Tropical Chia Pudding (page 52)	Black Bean and Mango Salad Stuffed Avocados (page 91)	Lemon-Caper Fish and Veggies en Papillote (page 108)
3	Leftover Zucchini Bread Baked Oatmeal	Leftover Easy Israeli Shrimp Salad	Leftover Sheet Pan Miso Honey Tempeh and Broccoli with Crispy Miso-Glazed Brussels Sprouts (page 143)
4	Leftover Tropical Chia Pudding	Leftover Black Bean and Mango Salad Stuffed Avocados	Bruschetta Branzino (page 114) with Garlicky Roasted Green Beans with Lemon (page 141)
5	Leftover Zucchini Bread Baked Oatmeal	Easy Israeli Shrimp Salad (page 61)	Roasted Red Pepper Rigatoni (page 87) with Simple Ratatouille (page 144)
6	Smoked Salmon Scramble (page 53)	Leftover Black Bean and Mango Salad Stuffed Avocados	Orange-Glazed Shrimp Stir-Fry (page 120)
7	Smoked Salmon Scramble (page 53)	Totally Loaded Sweet Potato Nachos (page 92)	Lentil "Meatballs" and Spaghetti (page 84)
Snacks and Sides	Spicy Popcorn Snack Mix (page 134) Coconut Brownie Energy Bites (page 136)		

Planning and Prepping

This week's recipes are approachable, simple, and nutritious, but don't skimp on flavor. Plus, most meals have some component that can be prepped in advance.

- For weekday breakfasts, you'll prepare two make-ahead meals. The Zucchini Bread Baked Oatmeal and Tropical Chia Pudding can both be made days in advance and stored in the refrigerator. In the morning, you can heat up the oatmeal before eating or enjoy it cold.

- The day before you start the meal plan, make the Israeli Shrimp Salad. There's no lettuce to get soggy, so I encourage you to prepare it in advance since it tastes better when it sits overnight. The salad will last two to three days in the refrigerator.

- On Day 1, make the salad for the Black Bean and Mango Salad Stuffed Avocados. Again, there's no lettuce to get soggy, which makes for a perfect salad to prep in advance.

- Prepare the Sheet Pan Miso Honey Tempeh and Broccoli on the day before you start on Day 1. If preparing in advance, undercook slightly (about 5 to 10 minutes) to account for time to reheat.

- Make the bruschetta for the Bruschetta Branzino a day or two in advance. Store in an airtight container to allow the flavors to meld for a day or two.

SHOPPING LIST

CANNED AND BOTTLED ITEMS

- ☐ Black beans, low-sodium (2 [15-ounce] cans)
- ☐ Broth, vegetable, low-sodium (1 [32-ounce] carton)
- ☐ Coconut milk, unsweetened (2 [13.5-ounce] cans)
- ☐ Marinara sauce (1 [28-ounce] jar)
- ☐ Salsa (1 [15.5-ounce] jar)
- ☐ Tomatoes, fire roasted, diced (1 [15-ounce] can)
- ☐ Tomato paste (1 [6-ounce] can)

DAIRY AND EGGS

- ☐ Butter, unsalted (1 stick)
- ☐ Cheddar cheese, shredded (4 ounces)
- ☐ Eggs, large (1 dozen)
- ☐ Milk, 2 percent (1 quart)
- ☐ Parmesan cheese, grated (1 ounce)
- ☐ Tempeh (1 [8-ounce] package)

SEAFOOD

- ☐ Branzino, with skin (4 [6-ounce] fillets)
- ☐ Smoked salmon (4 ounces)
- ☐ Shrimp, raw, peeled and deveined (2 pounds)
- ☐ White fish fillets like flounder, snapper, tilapia (4 [6-ounce] 1½-inch-thick fillets)

PANTRY ITEMS

Note that these items will be used throughout the meal plan, so be sure to keep them stocked throughout the month.

- ☐ Agave syrup
- ☐ Allspice, ground
- ☐ Anchovy paste
- ☐ Baking powder
- ☐ Basil, dried
- ☐ Bay leaves
- ☐ Black pepper, ground
- ☐ Bread crumbs, whole-wheat, panko
- ☐ Bread crumbs, whole-wheat, seasoned
- ☐ Brown sugar, light
- ☐ Capers
- ☐ Cayenne pepper, ground
- ☐ Chia seeds
- ☐ Chili powder
- ☐ Cinnamon, ground
- ☐ Cocoa powder, unsweetened
- ☐ Coconut, unsweetened, shredded
- ☐ Coffee grounds
- ☐ Cornstarch or all-purpose flour
- ☐ Cranberries, dried
- ☐ Cumin, ground
- ☐ Curry powder
- ☐ Fennel seeds
- ☐ Flaxseed, ground
- ☐ Flour, all-purpose
- ☐ Garlic powder
- ☐ Ginger, ground
- ☐ Honey
- ☐ Hot chili sauce, like sriracha
- ☐ Italian seasoning, dried

Continued >

- ☐ Ketchup
- ☐ Maple syrup
- ☐ Marmalade, orange
- ☐ Mayonnaise
- ☐ Miso paste, white
- ☐ Mustard, Dijon
- ☐ Nutritional yeast
- ☐ Oat flour
- ☐ Oats, old-fashioned, rolled
- ☐ Oats, quick-cooking
- ☐ Oil, avocado
- ☐ Oil, olive, extra-virgin
- ☐ Old Bay Seasoning
- ☐ Onion powder
- ☐ Oregano, dried
- ☐ Parsley, dried
- ☐ Pepitas
- ☐ Pepperoncini, jarred
- ☐ Prunes
- ☐ Raisins, golden
- ☐ Red pepper flakes
- ☐ Roasted red peppers, water-packed
- ☐ Salt
- ☐ Shredded coconut, unsweetened
- ☐ Smoked paprika
- ☐ Soy sauce, low-sodium
- ☐ Sugar, brown
- ☐ Sugar, granulated (optional)
- ☐ Sumac, ground
- ☐ Sunflower seed butter
- ☐ Sunflower seeds
- ☐ Thyme, dried
- ☐ Vanilla extract
- ☐ Vinegar, apple cider
- ☐ Vinegar, balsamic
- ☐ Vinegar, red wine
- ☐ Vinegar, rice
- ☐ Vinegar, white
- ☐ White pepper, ground
- ☐ Worcestershire sauce

PRODUCE

- ☐ Avocados (3)
- ☐ Basil, fresh (1 bunch)
- ☐ Bell pepper, red (4)
- ☐ Bell pepper, yellow (1)
- ☐ Broccoli, head (1)
- ☐ Brussels sprouts (1 pound)
- ☐ Chives, fresh (1 bunch)
- ☐ Cilantro, fresh (1 bunch)
- ☐ Cucumbers, Persian (6)
- ☐ Eggplant (1)
- ☐ Garlic (1 head)
- ☐ Ginger (1 knob)
- ☐ Green beans or haricot verts (2 pounds)

- [ ] Jalapeño (1) (optional)
- [ ] Lemons (5)
- [ ] Lime (2)
- [ ] Mango (2)
- [ ] Mushrooms, white button (1 pint)
- [ ] Onion, red (1)
- [ ] Onion, yellow (3)
- [ ] Orange (1)
- [ ] Parsley, fresh (1 bunch)
- [ ] Pineapple (1)
- [ ] Scallions (1 bunch)
- [ ] Sweet potatoes (4)
- [ ] Tomatoes, grape or cherry (2 pints)
- [ ] Zucchini (5)

OTHER

- [ ] Edamame, dry roasted (1 [4-ounce] bag)
- [ ] Lentils, green (1 cup)
- [ ] Pasta, rigatoni, penne, or gemelli (1 pound)
- [ ] Pasta, whole-wheat spaghetti (1 pound)
- [ ] Popcorn, air-popped (1 [4.4-ounce] bag)
- [ ] Whole-wheat bread (optional)
- [ ] Whole-grain O's cereal, such as Cheerios (1 [8.9-ounce] box)

THE SECOND WEEK

DAY	BREAKFAST	LUNCH	DINNER
8	Ricotta-Pear Toast with Maple-Roasted Pepitas (page 51)	Greek Hummus Collard Wraps (page 90)	Tuna Avocado Burgers (page 122) with Old Bay–Spiced Sweet Potato Wedges (page 142)
9	Tropical Chia Pudding (page 52)	Leftover Tuna Avocado Burgers	Hearty Black Bean Burgers with Honey-Pickled Red Onions (page 78)
10	Leftover Ricotta-Pear Toast with Maple-Roasted Pepitas	Leftover Hearty Black Bean Burgers with Honey-Pickled Red Onions over salad	Shredded Brussels Sprouts and Goat Cheese Flatbread (page 94)
11	Leftover Tropical Chia Pudding	Greek Hummus Collard Wraps (page 90)	Pepita Pesto–Crusted Cod (page 102)
12	Leftover Ricotta-Pear Toast with Maple-Roasted Pepitas	Butternut Squash and Lentil Soup (page 69)	Totally Loaded Sweet Potato Nachos (page 92)
13	Oat Flour Blueberry Pancakes (page 51)	Roasted Carrot and Apple Soup (page 70) with Shredded Brussels Sprouts and Apple Slaw with Cider-Mustard Dressing (page 62)	30-Minute Mussels Marinara (page 121) with arugula salad
14	Leftover Oat Flour Blueberry Pancakes	Leftover Butternut Squash and Lentil Soup	Healthy Baked Fish and Chips (page 116)
Snacks and Sides	Roasted Red Pepper White Bean Hummus and crudités (page 113) Five-Ingredient Portobello Pizzas (page 137)		

Planning and Prepping

This week's meal plan is rich in fall flavors, like butternut squash, pear, pumpkin, Brussels sprouts, and cranberries. It's also convenient. A few lunches use leftovers from the night before. To bulk up leftovers, add a veggie side, like a no-fuss salad.

- Tropical Chia Pudding will last in your refrigerator for four to five days, so prep it in advance for easy mornings.

- Make the Maple-Roasted Pepitas beforehand for a quick toast on alternate days.

- On Day 13, make the Oat Flour Blueberry Pancakes so you can just reheat and eat the next day. You can even double the recipe and freeze (once cooled) for next week's breakfast.

- Pickled onions stay fresh for a couple of weeks, so make those for the Hearty Black Bean Burgers with Honey-Pickled Red Onions when convenient.

- If you want to DIY the hummus instead of using store-bought for the Greek Hummus Collard Wraps, make the Roasted Red Pepper White Bean Hummus one to two days ahead. Leftovers are also great for snacking.

- Soups are best made ahead, since they typically take longer than 30 minutes to prep. Both the Butternut Squash and Lentil Soup and Roasted Carrot and Apple Soup can be made several days in advance and freeze well, too.

- Prepare salad dressings and sauces like the Pepita Pesto a few days in advance for quicker prep.

SHOPPING LIST

CANNED AND BOTTLED ITEMS

☐ Black beans, no added salt
(3 [15-ounce] cans)

☐ Broth, vegetable, low-sodium
(3 [32-ounce] cartons)

☐ Coconut milk, unsweetened
(2 [13.5-ounce] cans)

☐ Marinara sauce (1 [16-ounce] jar)

☐ Salsa (1 [15.5-ounce] jar)

☐ Tomatoes, crushed (2 [28-ounce] cans)

☐ Tuna, albacore, water-packed
(2 [5-ounce] cans)

☐ White cannellini beans
(1 [15-ounce] can)

DAIRY AND EGGS

☐ Butter, unsalted (1 stick)

☐ Cheddar cheese, shredded (4 ounces)

☐ Eggs, large (6)

☐ Feta cheese, crumbled (4 ounces)

☐ Goat cheese (4 ounces)

☐ Greek yogurt, plain, 2 percent
(8 ounces) (optional)

☐ Milk, 2 percent (1 quart)

☐ Mozzarella cheese (8 ounces)

☐ Parmesan cheese, grated (1 ounce)

☐ Ricotta cheese (1 [15-ounce] container)

SEAFOOD

☐ Cod (8 [6-ounce] 1-inch-thick fillets)

☐ Mussels (4 pounds)

PRODUCE

☐ Alfalfa sprouts (1 pint)

☐ Apples, McIntosh (3)

☐ Arugula (1 [5-ounce] bag)

☐ Avocado (2)

☐ Basil, fresh (5 bunches)

☐ Blueberries (1 pint)

☐ Brussels sprouts, shredded (3 pounds)

☐ Butternut squash (1 medium)

☐ Carrots (6 pounds)

☐ Celery (2 heads)

☐ Cilantro (1 bunch)

☐ Collard greens (2 bunches)

- ☐ Cucumber (1)
- ☐ Garlic (1 bulb)
- ☐ Mango (1)
- ☐ Mushrooms, portobello (8)
- ☐ Jalapeño (1) (optional)
- ☐ Jicama (1)
- ☐ Lettuce, butter (1 head)
- ☐ Lettuce, romaine (1 head)
- ☐ Onion, red (3)

- ☐ Onion, yellow (2)
- ☐ Parsley (1 bunch)
- ☐ Pear (2)
- ☐ Pineapple (1)
- ☐ Potatoes, baby gold (2 pounds)
- ☐ Scallions (1 bunch)
- ☐ Sweet potatoes (2 pounds)
- ☐ Tomato, large (1)

OTHER

- ☐ Hummus (1 [10-ounce] container)
- ☐ Lentils, green (1 cup)
- ☐ Naan, whole-wheat (4 pieces)
- ☐ Pasta, whole-wheat (8 ounces)

- ☐ Sprouted grain bread (1 loaf)
- ☐ White wine, dry (6 ounces)
- ☐ Whole-wheat buns (10)

THE THIRD WEEK

DAY	BREAKFAST	LUNCH	DINNER
15	Oat Flour Blueberry Pancakes (page 51)	Mason Jar Sushi Salad (page 112)	Sheet Pan Miso Honey Tempeh and Broccoli (page 86)
16	Smoked Trout Breakfast Salad (page 56)	Confetti Farro and Tuna Salad with Lime Vinaigrette (page 64)	Mushroom and Red Bean Tacos (page 80)
17	Zucchini Bread Baked Oatmeal (page 50)	10-Vegetable Soup (page 72) with Marinated Tofu Greek Salad (page 88)	Cajun-Spiced Snapper with Pineapple Salsa (page 118) with Garlicky Roasted Green Beans with Lemon (page 141)
18	Leftover Oat Flour Blueberry Pancakes	Leftover Confetti Farro and Tuna Salad with Lime Vinaigrette	Lentil Sloppy Joes with Tangy Cabbage Slaw (page 82)
19	Leftover Zucchini Bread Baked Oatmeal	Leftover 10-Vegetable Soup and leftover Marinated Tofu Greek Salad	Slow-Roasted Dijon Arctic Char (page 104) and Crispy Miso-Glazed Brussels Sprouts (page 143)
20	Smoked Salmon Scramble (page 53)	Leftover Confetti Farro and Tuna Salad with Lime Vinaigrette	Whole Roasted Cauliflower with Sunflower Seed Pesto (page 96) and leftover 10-Vegetable Soup
21	Leftover Zucchini Bread Baked Oatmeal	Zesty Crab and Avocado Bites (page 132) and Roasted Red Pepper White Bean Hummus (page 133) and crudités	Lentil "Meatballs" and Spaghetti (page 84) with Broccoli Caesar Salad with Hummus Caesar Dressing (page 68)
Snacks and Sides	Coconut Brownie Energy Bites (page 136) Simple Ratatouille (page 144)		

Planning and Prepping

Have you ever had a salad for breakfast? This week you'll try! Plus, a "snack lunch" and many make-ahead options are available.

- Simplify your mornings by making the Oat Flour Blueberry Pancakes and Zucchini Bread Baked Oatmeal in advance. You can freeze the pancakes and warm them in a toaster oven in the morning.

- Prep salad dressings a few days in advance for the Mason Jar Sushi Salad and Confetti Farro and Tuna Salad.

- Prep the ingredients for the 10-Vegetable Soup up to several days in advance. Freeze the soup in individual poritons for ease.

- Marinate the tofu the night before serving it in the Marinated Tofu Greek Salad.

- Prepare the Roasted Red Pepper White Bean Hummus up to two days in advance.

- Make the cabbage slaw for the Lentil Sloppy Joes with Tangy Cabbage Slaw and the pineapple salsa for the Cajun-Spiced Snapper a day in advance and store them in airtight containers in the refrigerator.

SHOPPING LIST

CANNED AND BOTTLED ITEMS

- ☐ Broth, vegetable, low-sodium (3 [32-ounce] cartons)
- ☐ Fire-roasted tomatoes, diced (1 [15-ounce] can)
- ☐ Hamburger buns, whole-wheat (4)
- ☐ Kidney beans (1 [15-ounce] cans)
- ☐ Marinara sauce (1 [28-ounce] jar)

- ☐ Tomatoes, crushed (1 [28-ounce] can)
- ☐ Tomato paste (1 [6-ounce] can)
- ☐ Tuna, albacore, olive oil-packed (2 [5-ounce] cans)
- ☐ White cannellini beans (2 [15-ounce] cans)

DAIRY AND EGGS

- ☐ Butter, unsalted (1 sticks)
- ☐ Eggs, large (2 dozen)
- ☐ Milk, 2-percent (1 quart)

- ☐ Parmesan cheese, grated (2 ounces)
- ☐ Parmesan cheese, shaved (1 ounce) (optional)
- ☐ Tempeh (1 [8-ounce] package)

SEAFOOD

- ☐ Arctic char (4 [6-ounce] fillets)
- ☐ Lump crabmeat (16 ounces)
- ☐ Smoked salmon (4 ounces)

- ☐ Smoked trout (8 ounces)
- ☐ Snapper (4 [6-ounce] fillets)

PRODUCE

- ☐ Arugula (2 [5-ounce] bags)
- ☐ Avocados (2)
- ☐ Basil, fresh (3 bunches)
- ☐ Beans, green (12 ounces)
- ☐ Beans, string (12 ounces)
- ☐ Bell pepper, green (1)

- ☐ Bell pepper, red (4)
- ☐ Blueberries (1 pint)
- ☐ Broccoli, large (2 heads)
- ☐ Brussels sprouts (1 pound)
- ☐ Cabbage, red (2 heads)
- ☐ Carrots (2 pounds)

- ☐ Carrots, shredded (1 [8-ounce] bag)
- ☐ Cauliflower, large (1 head)
- ☐ Celery (2 heads)
- ☐ Chives, fresh (1 bunch) (optional)
- ☐ Cilantro, fresh (1 bunch)
- ☐ Corn (2 ears)
- ☐ Cucumber, English (1)
- ☐ Dill, fresh (1 bunch)
- ☐ Eggplant, small (1)
- ☐ Garlic (1 bulb)
- ☐ Ginger (1 knob)
- ☐ Jalapeño (1)
- ☐ Jicama (1)
- ☐ Kale (2 large bunches)
- ☐ Leeks (1)
- ☐ Lemons (3)
- ☐ Limes (4)
- ☐ Mushrooms, sliced (1 pound)
- ☐ Onion, red (2)
- ☐ Onion, yellow (4)
- ☐ Pineapple (1)
- ☐ Scallions (1 bunch)
- ☐ Tomatoes, grape or cherry (1 pint)
- ☐ Zucchini (5)

FROZEN

- ☐ Edamame, shelled (1 [10-ounce] bag)

OTHER

- ☐ Bread, whole-wheat (1 loaf) (optional)
- ☐ Brown rice, short-grain (1 cup)
- ☐ Farro, pearled (½ cup)
- ☐ Hummus (1 [10-ounce] container)
- ☐ Lentils, green (1 cup)
- ☐ Seaweed sheets, nori (2)
- ☐ Spaghetti, whole-wheat (1 [1-pound] box)
- ☐ Tofu, extra firm (1 [14-ounce] block)
- ☐ Tortilla chips, corn, round (1 [8-ounce] bag)

THE FOURTH WEEK

DAY	BREAKFAST	LUNCH	DINNER
22	Tropical Chia Pudding (page 52)	Marinated Tofu Greek Salad (page 88)	Orange-Glazed Shrimp Stir-Fry (page 120)
23	Ricotta-Pear Toast with Maple-Roasted Pepitas (page 54)	Leftover Orange-Glazed Shrimp Stir-Fry and Shaved Fennel, Corn, and Peach Salad (page 60)	Sheet Pan Jerk Fish Tacos (page 100)
24	Leftover Tropical Chia Pudding	Marinated Tofu Greek Salad (page 88)	30-Minute Coconut Shrimp Curry (page 126)
25	Leftover Ricotta-Pear Toast with Maple-Roasted Pepitas	Black Bean and Mango Salad Stuffed Avocados (page 91)	No-Fuss Crab Cakes with Tzatziki Sauce (page 106)
26	Leftover Tropical Chia Pudding	Leftover No-Fuss Crab Cakes with Tzatziki Sauce and Shaved Fennel, Corn, and Peach Salad (page 60)	Roasted Red Pepper Rigatoni (page 87) and Broccoli Caesar Salad with Hummus Caesar Dressing (page 68)
27	Mexican-Style Shakshuka (page 57)	Leftover Black Bean and Mango Salad Stuffed Avocados	Lemon-Caper Fish and Veggies en Papillote (page 108)
28	Leftover Mexican-Style Shakshuka	Leftover Broccoli Caesar Salad with Hummus Caesar Dressing and Nut-Free Tuna Waldorf Salad Bites (page 135)	Grilled Scallop and Pineapple Skewers with Roasted Poblano Pepper Sauce (page 110)
Snacks and Sides	Mocha-Avocado Pudding (page 151) Raw Zoodle Salad with Avocado Miso Dressing (page 143)		

Planning and Prepping

By Week 4, you may have a better idea of how to save time in the kitchen during the week and what parts of recipes can be made in advance.

Here's what you can do over the weekend to make the week easier:

- Prepare Maple-Roasted Pepitas for the Ricotta-Pear Toast in advance. Leftovers make a great snack.

- Marinate the tofu on Day 21 for lunches throughout the week.

- Shave fennel using a mandolin for the Shaved Fennel, Corn, and Peach Salad one day before making.

- Chop the onions and peppers for the Jerk Fish Tacos one to two days in advance. Store in an airtight container in the refrigerator until use.

- Form crab cakes and make tzatziki sauce up to one day in advance. Wrap the crab cakes well and store in the refrigerator. Cook just before serving.

- Make roasted red pepper sauce for the rigatoni one to two days prior. Store in the refrigerator. Warm up on the stovetop while cooking the pasta.

- Prepare the Caesar dressing a few days in advance and store in the refrigerator.

- The roasted poblano sauce can be made one to two days in advance and stored in the refrigerator.

SHOPPING LIST

CANNED AND BOTTLED ITEMS

- ☐ Black beans, low-sodium (1 [15-ounce] can)

- ☐ Coconut milk, unsweetened, full-fat (3 [13.5-ounce] cans)

- ☐ Salsa (2 [15.5-ounce] jars)

- ☐ Tuna, water-packed (1 [5-ounce] can)

DAIRY AND EGGS

- ☐ Butter, unsalted (1 stick)

- ☐ Eggs, large (1 dozen)

- ☐ Greek yogurt, 2 percent (8 ounces)

- ☐ Parmesan cheese, grated (1 ounce)

- ☐ Ricotta cheese (1 [15-ounce] container)

Continued >

SEAFOOD

- ☐ Crabmeat, jumbo lump (8 ounces)
- ☐ Flounder (4 [6-ounce] fillets)
- ☐ Scallops (1 pound)
- ☐ Shrimp, raw, peeled and deveined (2 pounds)
- ☐ White fish: e.g., flounder, snapper, or tilapia (4 [6-ounce] 1½-inch-thick fillets)

PRODUCE

- ☐ Avocado (6)
- ☐ Bell pepper, red (4)
- ☐ Bell pepper, yellow (1)
- ☐ Broccoli (2 heads)
- ☐ Carrots, shredded (1 [8-ounce] bag)
- ☐ Cilantro, fresh (1 bunch)
- ☐ Corn, whole ears (2)
- ☐ Cucumber, English (3)
- ☐ Dill, fresh (2 bunches)
- ☐ Fennel (4 bulbs)
- ☐ Garlic (1 bulb)
- ☐ Grapes, red (1 bunch)
- ☐ Haricot verts (1 pound)
- ☐ Jalapeño (1)
- ☐ Lemons (5)
- ☐ Limes (5)
- ☐ Mangos (2)
- ☐ Mushrooms, white button (8 ounces)
- ☐ Onion, red, large (1)
- ☐ Onion, yellow (3)
- ☐ Orange (1)
- ☐ Parsley, fresh (2 bunches)
- ☐ Peaches (2)
- ☐ Pears (2)
- ☐ Pineapple (1)
- ☐ Poblano peppers (2)
- ☐ Scallions (1 bunch)
- ☐ Snap peas (8 ounces)
- ☐ Tomatoes, grape (1 pint)
- ☐ Zucchini (4)

OTHER

- ☐ Hummus (1 [10-ounce] container)
- ☐ Pasta, rigatoni, penne, or gemelli (1 [1-pound] box)
- ☐ Rice, brown (1 cup)
- ☐ Sprouted grain bread (1 loaf)
- ☐ Tofu, extra firm (1 [14-ounce] block)
- ☐ Tortillas, corn or whole-wheat (8)

BEYOND WEEK 4

After 28 days of following the pescatarian meal plan, you've officially adopted the pescatarian way of eating, and you're ready for the next step. If you feel a tad nervous about successfully following the fish-forward way of eating on your own, that's normal. But you're ready to embark on the pescatarian lifestyle.

As you know, the pescatarian diet is not restrictive in the way the word "diet" is typically used. It's a flexible lifestyle with a few guiding principles you've learned over the past 28 days. Remember, include fish and seafood as your primary animal protein. Choose plant-based proteins, like beans, lentils, nuts, and seeds. Eat the rainbow of vegetables you see at the market, and add healthy fats to fully reap the benefits of the pescatarian lifestyle. Choose fiber-filled whole-grains and starchy vegetables to balance your plate. Indulge in sweets and desserts occasionally, when the craving strikes.

It takes more than 28 days to adopt new habits and make lasting behavior changes, so keep practicing the pescatarian principles to reap the health benefits associated with this lifestyle. You'll have more energy, reduce your risk of chronic diseases, and effortlessly maintain a healthy weight for your body.

My number-one piece of advice to successfully adopt the pescatarian way of living is to continue planning. As I said earlier, "Proper planning provides for peak performance!" Create your own meal plans and shopping lists, even beyond the recipes found in this book, to stay organized and save money at the grocery store.

Even more, stock your pantry with the pescatarian essentials. Create a running list of pantry necessities you need to replenish at the supermarket. I suggest hanging a piece of paper on the inside of your pantry cabinet(s) (or keep a note on your phone) so you never forget to jot it down. Canned fish and beans are two pescatarian pantry staples you should always have to whip up a health-boosting meal in minutes.

Last, keep cooking simple. The recipes in this book are designed to be easy enough for new home cooks. Stressing about preparing pescatarian-friendly meals will only negate the health benefits you gain from this eating style. Stick to the cooking methods you find most approachable, and when in doubt, throw a piece of fish in a parchment paper packet to bake it en papillote. Alternatively, sear a fish fillet for just a few minutes on each side (depending on the thickness) and top with store-bought sauce. Sauté some shellfish with veggies to make a quick stir-fry or add tomato sauce for a primavera-style dish. Once you feel comfortable with these starter techniques, try poaching, grilling, or even cooking a whole fish. Before you know it, you'll be an expert!

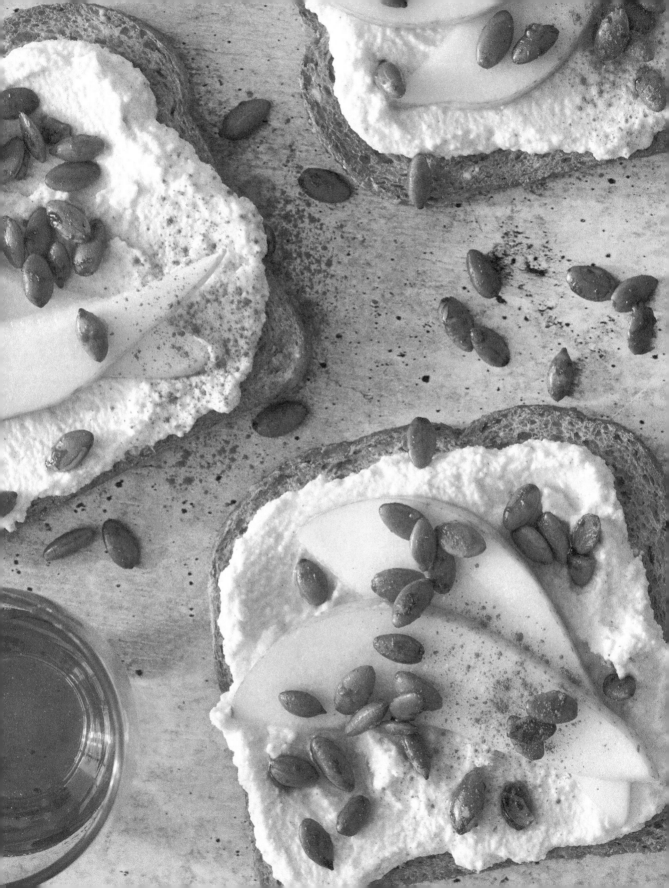

CHAPTER FOUR

BREAKFAST

ZUCCHINI BREAD BAKED OATMEAL

SERVES
4

PREP TIME:
5 minutes

COOK TIME:
25 minutes

30 MINUTES

GLUTEN-FREE

GF

HEART HEALTHY

VEGETARIAN

Baked oatmeal is a delicious and nutritious make-ahead breakfast. Oats are rich in soluble fiber called beta-glucan, which increases feelings of fullness and helps reduce blood sugar and cholesterol levels. I enjoy baked oatmeal with yogurt or a drizzle of sunflower seed butter for an extra protein boost.

2 cups rolled oats

¼ cup chia seeds

2 teaspoons ground cinnamon

1 teaspoon baking powder

½ teaspoon salt

1 cup low-fat milk

3 large eggs

2 tablespoons maple syrup (optional)

1 teaspoon vanilla extract

1 cup packed shredded zucchini, squeezed of excess water

½ cup golden raisins

1. Preheat the oven to 350°F. Line an 8-by-8-inch baking dish with parchment paper and set aside.

2. In a large bowl, mix the oats, chia seeds, cinnamon, baking powder, and salt.

3. Add the milk, eggs, maple syrup (if using), and vanilla. Mix until combined.

4. Gently fold in the zucchini and raisins.

5. Transfer the oat mixture to the prepared baking dish. Bake for 25 minutes, until the top and edges are golden brown.

6. Allow the baked oatmeal to cool completely before cutting into individual servings. Store in the refrigerator for up to 5 days.

Substitution Tip: Adding shredded zucchini is a great way to boost your veggie intake at breakfast, plus it keeps this baked oatmeal recipe extra moist. If zucchini is not in season, substitute shredded carrots or chopped apples instead.

PER SERVING: CALORIES: 380; TOTAL FAT: 12G; SATURATED FAT: 3G; CARBOHYDRATES: 57G; FIBER: 11G; PROTEIN: 15G; SODIUM: 381MG

OAT FLOUR BLUEBERRY PANCAKES

Boost the nutrients of traditional pancakes by using whole-grain oat flour. You can DIY by grinding old-fashioned rolled oats into flour-like consistency in a high-powered blender. About 1 cup of old-fashioned oats will yield the 1 cup of oat flour used in this recipe. Double or triple the batch of pancake batter to freeze leftovers for a quick weekday breakfast. Just reheat in a toaster oven or skillet.

SERVES
4

PREP TIME:
15 minutes

COOK TIME:
15 minutes

30 MINUTES

GLUTEN-FREE

GF

HEART HEALTHY

VEGETARIAN

1 cup oat flour

1 tablespoon granulated sugar (optional)

1½ teaspoons baking powder

½ teaspoon ground cinnamon

½ teaspoon salt

¾ cup low-fat milk or nondairy milk

2 large eggs

1 teaspoon vanilla extract

½ cup blueberries

1 to 2 tablespoons unsalted butter

Maple syrup, for serving (optional)

1. In a medium bowl, mix together the oat flour, sugar (if using), baking powder, cinnamon, and salt.

2. Add the milk, eggs, and vanilla, mixing until the batter is smooth.

3. Fold in the blueberries and let the batter sit for 5 minutes.

4. In a cast iron skillet, heat the butter over medium heat. When the pan is hot, add ⅓ cup batter to the skillet. Let cook for 3 minutes before carefully flipping and cooking for another 3 minutes.

5. Repeat until all batter is used. Top with maple syrup (if using) before serving.

Variation Tip: Oats are naturally gluten-free, but due to cross-contamination in the fields and processing, be sure to purchase certified gluten-free oats, if needed. Pair pancakes with a boost of protein, like Greek yogurt, for a well-balanced and filling meal.

PER SERVING: CALORIES: 199; TOTAL FAT: 7G; SATURATED FAT: 3G; CARBOHYDRATES: 25G; FIBER: 3G; PROTEIN: 8G; SODIUM: 368MG

TROPICAL CHIA PUDDING

SERVES
4

PREP TIME:
1 hour

DAIRY-FREE

GLUTEN-FREE

GF

HEART HEALTHY

VEGETARIAN

Chia seeds are a fun ingredient to add to your pantry because these tiny black seeds absorb up to nine times their weight in liquid, creating a pudding-like texture when soaked in milk. Not to mention they contain healthy fats, fiber, and plant-based protein, and are a healthy part of a well-balanced breakfast. Just grab a spoon and imagine you're eating this tropical chia pudding on a beach! You can use frozen fruit to save on prep time, too.

½ cup chia seeds
1½ teaspoons ground cinnamon
Heaping ¼ teaspoon salt
2 cups full-fat coconut milk

1 cup diced pineapple
½ cup diced mango
½ cup unsweetened
    shredded coconut

1. In a medium bowl, combine the chia seeds, cinnamon, and salt.

2. Mix in the coconut milk, scraping the bottom of the bowl to be sure the chia seeds are fully combined and do not clump together. Let sit for 5 minutes, then mix again, making sure all chia seeds are incorporated.

3. Stir in the pineapple, mango, and shredded coconut.

4. Cover and refrigerate for at least 45 minutes or overnight. Divide into individual portions before serving.

Variation Tip: Boost the protein of your chia pudding by mixing in your favorite protein powder, like marine collagen.

Leftovers Tip: Chia pudding will store well in the refrigerator for up to 4 days. Double the batch to enjoy all week long.

PER SERVING: CALORIES: 489; TOTAL FAT: 41G; SATURATED FAT: 30G; CARBOHYDRATES: 27G; FIBER: 13G; PROTEIN: 8G; SODIUM: 173MG

SMOKED SALMON SCRAMBLE

After visiting Seattle with my husband, these salmon scrambles became our weekend brunch of choice paired with crusty whole-grain bread. The key to making a fluffy scramble is to slowly push the eggs around your pan over low to medium heat. If you rush and make it over high heat, you won't get pillowy curds. Since smoked salmon is ready to eat, add it once the heat is turned off. It will warm from the heat of the eggs.

SERVES
4

PREP TIME:
5 minutes

COOK TIME:
10 minutes

30 MINUTES

GLUTEN-FREE
GF

6 large eggs

2 tablespoons low-fat milk

¼ teaspoon salt

⅛ teaspoon freshly ground black pepper

1 tablespoon unsalted butter

4 ounces smoked salmon, chopped

Chopped fresh chives, for garnish (optional)

Whole-wheat bread, for serving (optional)

1. In a medium bowl, whisk the eggs, milk, salt, and pepper.

2. In an 8-inch nonstick skillet, heat the butter over low-medium heat.

3. When the butter has melted, add the egg mixture. As the eggs begin to set, using a spatula, gently push the eggs towards the center of the pan, forming soft, fluffy curds. Repeat until the eggs are nearly cooked through and no liquid remains, about 7 minutes. Turn off the heat.

4. Add in the smoked salmon, gently tossing around the pan. Sprinkle with chives (if using) before serving hot with whole-wheat toast (if using).

Variation Tip: Make a dairy-free smoked salmon scramble by using unflavored dairy-free milk or omitting the milk altogether. Substitute oil for the butter.

PER SERVING: CALORIES: 169; TOTAL FAT: 12G; SATURATED FAT: 5G; CARBOHYDRATES: 1G; FIBER: 0G; PROTEIN: 15G; SODIUM: 743MG

RICOTTA-PEAR TOAST WITH MAPLE-ROASTED PEPITAS

SERVES
4

PREP TIME:
10 Minutes

COOK TIME:
20 Minutes

30 MINUTES

(30)

VEGETARIAN

Toast is a blank canvas, full of opportunity. This fall-inspired creation is deliciously simple—with a touch of elegance, thanks to the maple-roasted pepitas. Opt for sprouted whole-grain bread for a boost of fiber and protein. Plus, the sprouting process makes grains more easily digestible.

FOR THE MAPLE-ROASTED PEPITAS

½ tablespoon maple syrup
½ tablespoon extra-virgin olive oil
1 teaspoon ground cinnamon

½ teaspoon salt
½ cup pepitas

FOR THE RICOTTA-PEAR TOAST

8 slices sprouted grain bread
1 cup ricotta cheese
1 teaspoon ground cinnamon

Heaping ⅛ teaspoon salt
1 large pear, thinly sliced

TO MAKE THE MAPLE-ROASTED PEPITAS

1. Preheat the oven to 325°F. Line a sheet pan with parchment paper and set aside.

2. In a medium bowl, mix together the maple syrup, olive oil, cinnamon, and salt.

3. Add the pepitas and mix until evenly coated.

4. Spread the pepitas on a parchment paper–lined sheet pan. Bake for 15 to 20 minutes, until lightly browned, being careful not to burn them.

5. Remove from the oven and allow pepitas to cool slightly.

1. Toast the bread to desired doneness.

2. While the bread is toasting, in a small bowl, combine the ricotta cheese, cinnamon, and salt.

3. Spread the ricotta mixture on the toasted bread. Top each toast with 1 to 2 slices of pear. Sprinkle the maple pepitas on top.

Leftovers Tip: Maple-roasted pepitas make a great snack. Let them cool completely, then add to an on-the-go container for a snack with healthy fats and protein any time!

PER SERVING: CALORIES: 390; TOTAL FAT: 16G; SATURATED FAT: 5G; CARBOHYDRATES: 50G; FIBER: 6G; PROTEIN: 17G; SODIUM: 692MG

SMOKED TROUT BREAKFAST SALAD

SERVES
4

PREP TIME:
10 minutes

COOK TIME:
20 minutes

30 MINUTES

DAIRY-FREE

GLUTEN-FREE
GF

Enjoy a bowl of salty smoked trout paired with spicy arugula, and juxtaposed with a silky yolk dressing, to start your day with a hefty dose of nutrients. For the optimal yolk ooze, it takes practice to learn how to poach an egg, but remember, practice makes perfect! Vinegar is the secret ingredient, as it helps the proteins in the egg white coagulate for a foolproof poach.

8 cups baby arugula

1½ tablespoons extra-virgin olive oil

Pinch salt

4 large eggs

1 teaspoon white vinegar

8 ounces smoked trout

Freshly ground black pepper

1. In a large bowl, toss the arugula, olive oil, and salt. Set aside.

2. Crack an egg into a ramekin or small saucer and set aside. Bring a small saucepan of water to a boil, then reduce the heat to a simmer. Add the vinegar to the water. Swirl the water with a knife, creating a vortex. Slip the egg into the water. Let cook, without touching the egg or water, for about 5 minutes, until the egg white is set. Using a slotted spoon, remove the egg from the water and drain on a paper towel. Be sure the water remains at a simmer as you repeat with the remaining eggs.

3. Distribute the arugula among four bowls. Divide the smoked trout among the bowls. Top each with a poached egg and pepper to taste.

Substitution Tip: Can't get the perfect poach down? No problem! Substitute eggs cooked over easy, medium, hard, or even scrambled instead.

PER SERVING: CALORIES: 205; TOTAL FAT: 13G; SATURATED FAT: 2G; CARBOHYDRATES: 2G; FIBER: 1G; PROTEIN: 20G; SODIUM: 120MG

MEXICAN-STYLE SHAKSHUKA

Shakshuka is a Middle Eastern breakfast dish of eggs poached in tomato sauce that I first fell in love with when I lived in Israel. Typically made with Mediterranean flavors, this Mexican-inspired twist uses jarred salsa to impart tons of flavor without skimping on nutrition. Cooked tomatoes are packed with the antioxidant lycopene. Check the ingredient list to choose a jarred salsa with no added sugar. This dish is best served fresh.

2 (15.5-ounce) jars salsa
8 large eggs
¼ cup coarsely chopped fresh cilantro

Freshly ground black pepper
Crusty whole-wheat bread, for serving (optional)

1. Preheat the oven to 375°F.

2. In a large oven-safe skillet or sauté pan, heat the salsa over medium heat for about 3 minutes, until simmering.

3. Create a small well in the salsa, towards the edge of the pan, and crack an egg into it. Spoon some salsa over the egg to prevent the white from spreading all over the pan. Repeat with remaining eggs throughout the skillet.

4. Transfer the skillet to the oven and bake for about 10 minutes, until the whites are mostly set. Keep in mind the eggs will continue to cook once you remove the skillet from the oven. The yolks will be runny; cook longer if you prefer a set yolk.

5. Top with cilantro and pepper before serving with crusty whole-wheat bread (if using).

Substitution Tip: Make shakshuka with more traditional flavors by using jarred tomato or marinara sauce, preferably with no added sugar. Top with parsley and oregano instead of cilantro.

PER SERVING: CALORIES: 205; TOTAL FAT: 10G; SATURATED FAT: 3G; CARBOHYDRATES: 15G; FIBER: 4G; PROTEIN: 16G; SODIUM: 1032MG

SERVES
4

PREP TIME:
5 minutes

COOK TIME:
15 minutes

30 MINUTES

DAIRY-FREE

GLUTEN-FREE
GF

HEART HEALTHY

VEGETARIAN

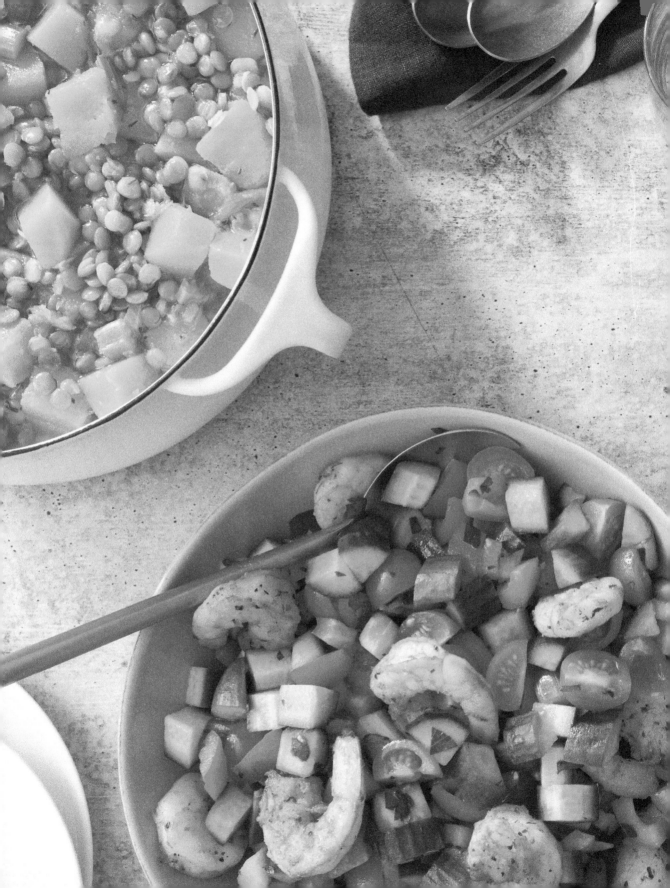

SHAVED FENNEL, CORN, AND PEACH SALAD

SERVES
4

PREP TIME:
10 minutes

30 MINUTES

DAIRY-FREE

GLUTEN-FREE

GF

HEART HEALTHY

VEGETARIAN

This lettuce-less medley is a great way to beat salad boredom with fennel. Fennel has a slightly sweet licorice-like flavor and is packed with antioxidants and fiber. This summery combination pairs great with seafood, making it the perfect side for many dishes throughout the book.

4 cups shaved or thinly sliced fennel

1 cup raw corn kernels (fresh or frozen and thawed)

2 medium peaches, thinly sliced

1 avocado, sliced

¼ cup chopped fresh cilantro

¼ teaspoon red pepper flakes

2 tablespoons extra-virgin olive oil

⅛ teaspoon sea salt

⅛ teaspoon freshly ground black pepper

1. In a large bowl, mix the fennel, corn, peaches, avocado, cilantro, and red pepper flakes.

2. Drizzle with olive oil and sprinkle the salt and pepper over the salad. Toss together. The salad will stay fresh in the refrigerator for 2 to 3 days.

Variation Tip: Adapt this side salad to a complete meal by adding a protein. Grilled fish or flaked wild canned salmon work great, but so do black beans, chickpeas, or lentils for a plant-based version.

PER SERVING: CALORIES: 162; TOTAL FAT: 8G; SATURATED FAT: 1G; CARBOHYDRATES: 24G; FIBER: 8G; PROTEIN: 4G; SODIUM: 429MG

EASY ISRAELI SHRIMP SALAD

After living in Israel for two years, I became obsessed with Israeli salad—even for breakfast! It's refreshing and satisfying and tastes even better the next day.

SERVES
4

PREP TIME:
20 minutes

COOK TIME:
6 minutes

30 MINUTES

DAIRY-FREE

GLUTEN-FREE
GF

HEART HEALTHY

FOR THE SALAD

3 cups chopped cucumbers
(6 Persian cucumbers)

1 red bell pepper, chopped

1½ cups chopped grape or cherry tomatoes

¼ cup coarsely chopped fresh parsley

1 tablespoon extra-virgin olive oil

¼ teaspoon sea salt

FOR THE SHRIMP

1 pound raw shrimp, peeled and deveined

¼ teaspoon salt

¼ teaspoon freshly ground black pepper

¼ teaspoon smoked paprika

¼ teaspoon dried oregano

¼ teaspoon garlic powder

1 tablespoon extra-virgin olive oil

TO MAKE THE SALAD

In a large bowl, toss the cucumbers, peppers, tomatoes, parsley, olive oil, and salt. Set aside.

TO MAKE THE SHRIMP

1. In a large bowl, season the shrimp with salt, pepper, smoked paprika, oregano, and garlic powder.

2. In a large skillet, warm the olive oil over medium heat. Add the shrimp to the pan and cook for 2 to 3 minutes on each side, or until shrimp are opaque. Transfer to a plate to cool.

3. Before serving, add the shrimp to the salad and toss together.

Variation Tip: Make this salad vegetarian by using chickpeas instead of shrimp.

PER SERVING: CALORIES: 196; TOTAL FAT: 8G; SATURATED FAT: 1G; CARBOHYDRATES: 8G; FIBER: 2G; PROTEIN: 25G; SODIUM: 402MG

SHREDDED BRUSSELS SPROUTS AND APPLE SLAW WITH CIDER-MUSTARD DRESSING

SERVES
4 to 6

PREP TIME:
15 minutes,
plus 15 minutes
to marinate

30 MINUTES

DAIRY-FREE

GLUTEN-FREE

GF

HEART HEALTHY

VEGETARIAN

With a base of shredded Brussels sprouts instead of lettuce, this is a must-try if you're in a salad rut. It's dotted with crunchy apple slices and sweet red onion, then dressed in a fall-inspired dressing. Plus, sturdy Brussels sprout leaves hold up well to the cider-mustard dressing, so it's great to pack for lunch on the go.

FOR THE SALAD

4 cups shredded Brussels sprouts

1 apple, cut into matchsticks (about 1 cup)

½ cup chopped red onion

FOR THE CIDER MUSTARD DRESSING

2 tablespoons Dijon mustard

2 tablespoons apple cider vinegar

2 tablespoons extra-virgin olive oil

1 teaspoon maple syrup

¼ teaspoon salt

⅛ teaspoon freshly ground black pepper

In a large bowl, combine the shredded Brussels sprouts, apple, and red onion. Set aside.

1. In a small bowl, mix together the Dijon, apple cider vinegar, olive oil, maple syrup, salt, and pepper until a uniform consistency forms. Alternatively, add all the ingredients to a mason jar with a lid and shake well.

2. Pour the dressing over the salad and mix together well. Refrigerate for at least 15 minutes before serving.

Variation Tip: Transform this side salad or leftovers into a complete and balanced meal by adding your favorite protein on top. Try grilled salmon or shrimp, chickpeas, or lentils.

PER SERVING: CALORIES: 144; TOTAL FAT: 8G; SATURATED FAT: 1G; CARBOHYDRATES: 19G; FIBER: 5G; PROTEIN: 4G; SODIUM: 260 MG

CONFETTI FARRO AND TUNA SALAD WITH LIME VINAIGRETTE

SERVES
4

PREP TIME:
15 minutes,
plus 30 to
45 minutes
cooling time

COOK TIME:
25 minutes

DAIRY-FREE

HEART HEALTHY

Nutty and slightly chewy farro is a whole grain packed with nearly 4 grams of fiber per serving. Layered with a rainbow of vegetables and convenient protein, this well-rounded salad is a packable lunch, perfect for a picnic, or your next potluck. Using pearled farro (versus whole farro) cuts down on prep time, since it cooks much faster.

FOR THE LIME VINAIGRETTE

¼ cup finely chopped fresh cilantro

¼ cup freshly squeezed lime juice

3 tablespoons extra-virgin olive oil

2 tablespoons honey

Scant ¼ teaspoon salt

⅛ teaspoon freshly ground black pepper

FOR THE CONFETTI FARRO

½ cup pearled farro

¼ teaspoon salt

4 cups shredded red cabbage

1 cup shredded carrots

½ cup chopped scallions, both white and green parts

1 red bell pepper, julienned

1 cup fresh corn kernels

2 (5-ounce) cans oil-packed white albacore tuna, drained

¼ teaspoon freshly ground black pepper

In a container or jar with a lid, muddle the cilantro leaves with the lime juice and olive oil. Mix in the honey. Season with the salt and pepper. Cover and shake to combine. Set aside.

TO MAKE THE CONFETTI FARRO

1. In a medium saucepan, combine 1 cup of water, farro, and salt. Bring to a boil, then reduce heat to low to simmer. Cover and cook for about 15 minutes, until all water is absorbed. Turn off the heat and let it sit covered for another 10 minutes.

2. While the farro cooks, in a large mixing bowl, combine the cabbage, carrots, scallions, bell pepper, and corn. Set aside.

3. When the farro is done cooking, let cool completely. Once cooled, add to the bowl with vegetables. Flake in the tuna and toss together with dressing. Season with pepper.

Substitution Tip: While farro adds great chewy texture to this salad, you can easily substitute any whole-grain you have available in your pantry. Try quinoa, bulgur, kamut, barley, or even whole-wheat pasta for a slight twist.

PER SERVING: CALORIES: 364; TOTAL FAT: 15G; SATURATED FAT: 3G; CARBOHYDRATES: 41G; FIBER: 6G; PROTEIN: 21G; SODIUM: 590MG

ROASTED VEGETABLE PANZANELLA SALAD

SERVES
4 to 6

PREP TIME:
20 minutes

COOK TIME:
40 minutes

DAIRY-FREE

HEART HEALTHY

VEGETARIAN

Roasting vegetables caramelizes their natural sugars, making them sweeter. Be sure not to overcrowd your sheet pans when roasting to avoid steaming the vegetables instead of roasting them. If necessary, use multiple sheet pans to ensure a delicious outcome. Also, keep cooking times in mind when roasting various vegetables together. For example, Brussels sprouts take longer to roast than butternut squash, so cut them into smaller pieces to quicken the cooking time.

2 large beets, peeled and chopped

2 cups halved Brussels sprouts

1 cup cubed peeled butternut squash

1 cup chopped carrots

1 large red onion, cut into eighths

4 tablespoons extra-virgin olive oil, divided

¾ teaspoon salt, divided

½ teaspoon freshly ground black pepper, divided

2 tablespoons balsamic vinegar

1 tablespoon Dijon mustard

1 tablespoon maple syrup or honey

3 cups cubed stale French bread

1. Preheat the oven to 375°F.

2. In a large bowl, toss the beets, Brussels sprouts, butternut squash, carrots, and red onion in 2 tablespoons of olive oil.

3. Transfer the vegetables to a large sheet pan. Sprinkle with ½ teaspoon of salt and ¼ teaspoon of pepper.

4. Roast for 40 minutes, tossing halfway through. The vegetables should be fork-tender and browned at edges when done cooking.

5. While the vegetables are roasting, in a small bowl, whisk the remaining 2 tablespoons olive oil, balsamic vinegar, Dijon, maple syrup, remaining ¼ teaspoon of salt and remaining ¼ teaspoon of pepper. Set aside.

6. When the vegetables are done roasting, transfer them to a large mixing bowl. Toss together with French bread and dressing. Let them sit for about 5 minutes before serving. Serve warm or at room temperature.

Substitution Tip: Use any crusty, stale bread instead of French bread. Crusty pumpernickel or rye bread would be delicious and add a punch of flavor, too. Alternatively, you could crumble up some crackers.

PER SERVING: CALORIES: 290; TOTAL FAT: 15G; SATURATED FAT: 2G; CARBOHYDRATES: 37G; FIBER: 6G; PROTEIN: 6G; SODIUM: 711MG

BROCCOLI CAESAR SALAD WITH HUMMUS CAESAR DRESSING

SERVES
4 to 6

PREP TIME:
15 minutes

30 MINUTES

DAIRY-FREE

GLUTEN-FREE

GF

HEART HEALTHY

This is a fun twist on the traditional Caesar salad with a velvety hummus-based dressing packed with garlicky flavor. Broccoli is loaded with vitamins and minerals, including vitamins A, C, and K; potassium; calcium; iron; and magnesium. The recipe calls for raw broccoli, but you can blanch the broccoli for a softer bite, if you'd like.

¼ cup hummus

Juice from 1 lemon

1 teaspoon anchovy paste

1 teaspoon Dijon mustard

½ tablespoon finely chopped garlic

Heaping ⅛ teaspoon sea salt

⅛ teaspoon freshly ground black pepper

1 large broccoli head, cut into small florets and stems peeled and chopped

¼ cup grated Parmesan cheese

1. In a large bowl, mix together the hummus, lemon juice, anchovy paste, Dijon, garlic, salt, and pepper.

2. Add the broccoli florets. Toss together so the broccoli is thoroughly coated in the dressing. Let sit for at least 10 minutes or up to 3 hours to allow the flavors to marinate.

3. Sprinkle the Parmesan cheese on top before serving.

Variation Tip: Not a fan of anchovy paste? Leave it out, but increase the amount of salt you add to the dressing.

Leftovers Tip: Double the dressing recipe and store in an airtight container in the refrigerator to slather on greens or use as a dip throughout the week.

PER SERVING: CALORIES: 103; TOTAL FAT: 5G; SATURATED FAT: 1G; CARBOHYDRATES: 12G; FIBER: 5G; PROTEIN: 8G; SODIUM: 279MG

BUTTERNUT SQUASH AND LENTIL SOUP

This hearty and filling butternut squash and lentil soup is a well-balanced meal, packed with plant-based protein, fiber, and healthy fats. With minimal hands-on time, this is a great make-ahead meal to enjoy all week for lunch, snack, or dinner.

SERVES
6 to 8

PREP TIME:
15 minutes

COOK TIME:
1 hour

DAIRY-FREE

GLUTEN-FREE
GF

HEART HEALTHY

VEGETARIAN

1 tablespoon extra-virgin olive oil

1 cup chopped yellow onion

1 cup chopped celery

2 garlic cloves, grated or finely chopped

4 cups cubed butternut squash (about 1 medium butternut squash)

½ teaspoon dried thyme

½ teaspoon salt

¼ teaspoon ground cumin

¼ teaspoon freshly ground black pepper

6 cups low-sodium vegetable stock

1 cup green lentils

2 bay leaves

1. In a large stock pot, heat the olive oil over medium heat. Sauté the onion, celery, and garlic for about 5 minutes, until the vegetables begin to soften and are almost translucent.

2. Mix in the butternut squash, thyme, salt, cumin, and pepper, continuing to sauté for about 15 minutes, until the squash is fork-tender.

3. Add the vegetable stock, lentils, and bay leaves.

4. Bring the mixture to a boil and then reduce to simmer and let cook for 30 minutes, or until lentils are completely cooked and soft.

5. Remove the bay leaves before serving warm.

Leftovers Tip: The soup will keep, refrigerated, for about a week. To freeze, store it in individual serving containers for up to 6 months.

PER SERVING: CALORIES: 208; TOTAL FAT: 3G; SATURATED FAT: 0G; CARBOHYDRATES: 37G; FIBER: 13G; PROTEIN: 11G; SODIUM: 354MG

ROASTED CARROT AND APPLE SOUP

With a hint of sweetness and a kick of spice, this creamy carrot and apple soup will warm you up with a hefty dose of beta-carotene to aid your immunity and vision. Pair a bowl with your favorite sandwich for a hearty and filling lunch, thanks to all the fiber from the carrots and apples. You can easily make in advance and freeze in individual portions to enjoy all winter long.

5 pounds carrots, chopped

2 McIntosh apples, sliced

¾ cup sliced red onion

3 tablespoons extra-virgin olive oil, divided

6 cups low-sodium vegetable broth or stock, plus more if needed

½ teaspoon red pepper flakes

½ teaspoon ground cinnamon

½ teaspoon dried oregano

½ teaspoon ground ginger

½ teaspoon salt

¼ teaspoon fennel seeds

¼ teaspoon freshly ground black pepper

Toasted pepitas, for serving (optional)

Plain Greek yogurt or coconut yogurt, for serving (optional)

1. Preheat the oven to 375°F.

2. On a large sheet pan, arrange the carrots, apples, and onion. Do not overcrowd the sheet; use more than one if needed. Toss with 2 tablespoons olive oil to evenly coat. Roast for 40 minutes, until fork-tender, tossing once halfway through roasting.

3. Remove from the oven and transfer to a large stock pot along with the vegetable broth, red pepper flakes, cinnamon, oregano, ginger, salt, fennel, and pepper. Using an immersion blender, blend until smooth. Alternatively, you can add the roasted vegetables and apples to a high-speed blender with the vegetable broth to blend until smooth.

4. Add more vegetable broth to obtain the desired consistency.

5. Bring the soup to a boil. Serve warm topped with toasted pepitas (if using) or yogurt (if using).

Substitution Tip: Carrots impart a good balance of sweet and earthy flavor to this soup, but you can use nearly any orange fall vegetable in this recipe. Butternut squash, acorn squash, and sweet potatoes all work well.

PER SERVING: CALORIES: 276; TOTAL FAT: 7G; SATURATED FAT: 1G; CARBOHYDRATES: 50G; FIBER: 12G; PROTEIN: 6G; SODIUM: 526MG

10-VEGETABLE SOUP

SERVES
8

PREP TIME:
15 minutes

COOK TIME:
45 minutes

DAIRY-FREE

GLUTEN-FREE

GF

HEART HEALTHY

VEGETARIAN

As soon as the weather starts to chill, my mom always has a big pot of this soup on the stove to warm up and prevent any pesky colds, since it's packed with vitamins and minerals. If you've never made soup before, this recipe is a perfect recipe to start with since it's hard to mess up. Leftovers are even better than a fresh bowl, so if possible, make a pot in advance for optimal flavor.

2 tablespoons extra-virgin olive oil

1 large yellow onion, chopped

¾ cup chopped carrots

½ cup chopped celery

1 teaspoon salt, divided

1 teaspoon freshly ground black pepper, divided

3 cups sliced mushrooms

2 cups chopped zucchini

1 red bell pepper, chopped

½ cup sliced leeks

½ cup roughly chopped string beans

1 (28-ounce) can crushed tomatoes

1 (15-ounce) can cannellini (white) beans, drained and rinsed

1 tablespoon balsamic vinegar

1 tablespoon Italian seasoning

8 cups low-sodium vegetable broth

6 cups roughly chopped kale

Shaved Parmesan cheese, for serving (optional, but recommended)

1. In a large stock pot, heat the olive oil over medium heat. Sauté the onions, carrots, and celery for about 5 minutes, or until softened. Season with ½ teaspoon of salt and ½ teaspoon of pepper.

2. Add the mushrooms, zucchini, bell pepper, leeks, and string beans and sauté for about 5 minutes, or until softened.

3. Mix in the crushed tomatoes, beans, balsamic vinegar, and Italian seasoning.

4. Add the broth and bring to a boil, then reduce to a simmer. Let the soup simmer for about 10 minutes before adding the kale. Cover and continue to simmer for 20 minutes.

5. Serve, topped with Parmesan cheese (if using).

Substitution Tip: This 10-Vegetable Soup is the perfect recipe to make with vegetables on their last lifeline before spoiling. Customize this recipe using whatever vegetables and beans you have on hand. Try shredded cabbage, spinach, Brussels sprouts, parsnips, eggplant, chickpeas, red beans, and more.

PER SERVING: CALORIES: 188; TOTAL FAT: 5G; SATURATED FAT: 1G; CARBOHYDRATES: 28G; FIBER: 8G; PROTEIN: 10G; SODIUM: 608MG

CAULIFLOWER CLAM CHOWDER

SERVES
6 to 8

PREP TIME:
20 minutes

COOK TIME:
50 minutes

Cauliflower clam chowder is a lighter version of the New England favorite. Creamy puréed cauliflower thickens the soup, with a hefty dose of vitamins, minerals, and fiber in place of heavy cream. I used canned clams for added convenience and a stronger punch of flavor from the clam juice. You can alternatively use 1½ cups clam juice and add chopped cooked clams.

2 tablespoons unsalted butter

½ cup chopped yellow onion

1 teaspoon finely minced garlic

2 tablespoons flour

6 cups small cauliflower florets (about ¾ cauliflower head)

4 cups low-sodium vegetable broth

2 (10-ounce) cans clams, juices separated and reserved (approximately 1½ cups juice)

1½ cups quartered baby gold potatoes

1 cup low-fat milk

2 bay leaves

½ teaspoon smoked paprika

½ teaspoon freshly ground black pepper

¼ teaspoon salt

1 tablespoon finely chopped parsley

1. In a large stock pot, melt the butter over medium heat. Cook the onions and garlic for about 2 minutes, stirring constantly, until fragrant.

2. Turn the heat to low, then whisk in the flour and cook for 1 to 2 minutes, until lightly browned.

3. Add the cauliflower, vegetable broth, the juice of the clams, potatoes, milk, bay leaves, smoked paprika, pepper, and salt. Mix until combined.

4. Bring to a boil, then reduce the heat to simmer. Cover and cook for 20 minutes, stirring occasionally.

5. Once the cauliflower and potatoes are fork-tender, remove the bay leaves and use an immersion blender to blend on low until the desired consistency forms. The soup should be chunky. Alternatively, transfer the contents of the pot to a blender to blend on low.

6. Simmer on low for 15 minutes to thicken.

7. Add the clams to the soup. Garnish with parsley before serving.

Variation Tip: This recipe can easily be made allergy friendly. To make it gluten-free, use gluten-free flour. To make it dairy-free, use nondairy butter and milk.

PER SERVING: CALORIES: 157; TOTAL FAT: 5G; SATURATED FAT: 3G; CARBOHYDRATES: 13G; FIBER: 3G; PROTEIN: 15G; SODIUM: 261MG

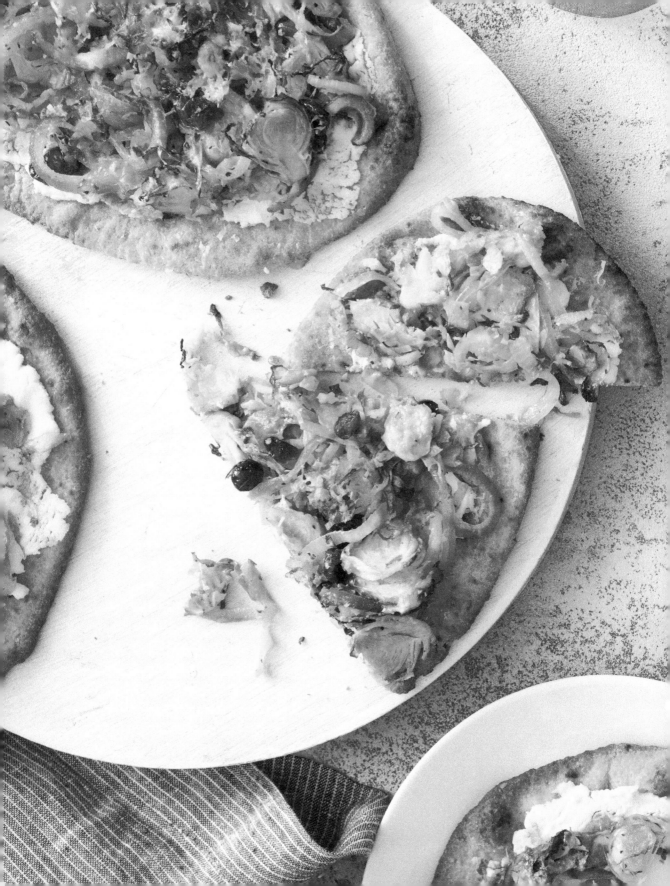

CHAPTER SIX

VEGETARIAN MAINS

HEARTY BLACK BEAN BURGERS WITH HONEY-PICKLED RED ONIONS

SERVES
6

PREP TIME:
20 minutes,
plus 15 minutes
refrigeration
time

COOK TIME:
20 minutes

DAIRY-FREE

HEART HEALTHY

VEGETARIAN

These flavorful and filling black bean burgers will become a go-to meat-free meal that even carnivores will enjoy! Plus, beans are a good source of fiber and protein that will help you stay full for hours. Serve like a traditional burger on a whole-wheat bun, or opt for a lighter meal and enjoy these burgers over a bed of greens. Either way, don't forget the quick-pickled onions for a bright burst of flavor with every bite!

FOR THE HONEY-PICKLED ONIONS

½ cup apple cider vinegar

¼ cup red wine vinegar

1 teaspoon sea salt

1 tablespoon honey

1 large red onion, very thinly sliced (about 2 cups)

FOR THE BLACK BEAN BURGERS

2 (15-ounce) cans low-sodium black beans, drained and rinsed, divided

¼ cup jarred salsa

1 large egg

2 garlic cloves, peeled

2 teaspoons ground cumin

1 teaspoon chili powder

1 teaspoon smoked paprika

1 teaspoon red pepper flakes

½ teaspoon salt

½ teaspoon freshly ground black pepper

½ cup quick oats

Whole-wheat buns, for serving

Butter lettuce leaves, for serving (optional)

Tomato slices, for serving (optional)

Avocado, for serving (optional)

Salsa, for serving (optional)

In a large jar, combine the apple cider vinegar, red wine vinegar, salt, and honey. Shake to combine. Add the onion. Let sit, occasionally shaking to combine, for at least 30 minutes or up to 4 hours.

TO MAKE THE BLACK BEAN BURGERS

1. In a food processor or high-speed blender, combine 1 can of black beans, the salsa, egg, garlic, cumin, chili powder, smoked paprika, red pepper flakes, salt, and pepper. Process until well combined. If you do not have a food processor, you could mash the beans with a fork, whisk the egg, and finely chop the garlic, then mix together with the spices to combine.

2. Transfer to a large bowl. Mix in the oats and the remaining can of beans. Cover and refrigerate for at least 15 minutes.

3. When ready to cook, preheat the oven to 375°F. Line a large sheet pan with parchment paper.

4. Form into patties, about one-half cup each. Gently flatten them with the palm of your hand on the sheet pan.

5. Bake for 15 minutes, then remove from the oven and carefully flip them. Return them to the oven for an additional 5 minutes. Alternatively, coat a cast iron pan with oil and cook the patties over medium-high heat for 5 to 7 minutes on each side.

6. Serve the burgers on buns with pickled onions, lettuce, tomato, avocado, and salsa.

Recipe Tip: Make it vegan by using a flax egg. Combine 1 tablespoon ground flaxseed with 3 tablespoons warm water in a small bowl. Mix to combine. Let sit for 10 minutes before adding to the recipe in place of the egg.

PER SERVING: CALORIES: 185; TOTAL FAT: 2G; SATURATED FAT: 1G; CARBOHYDRATES: 31G; FIBER: 9G; PROTEIN: 10G; SODIUM: 603MG

MUSHROOM AND RED BEAN TACOS

SERVES
4

PREP TIME:
5 minutes

COOK TIME:
15 minutes

30 MINUTES

DAIRY-FREE

HEART HEALTHY

VEGETARIAN

Hearty mushrooms are a perfect plant-based taco filling that delivers on flavor and texture while being low in fat. Mushrooms are more than 90 percent water, which escapes when cooking, so they will steam in an overcrowded pan. To avoid this, be sure to give the mushrooms enough room to brown and caramelize for optimal flavor.

½ tablespoon extra-virgin olive oil

2 pints sliced white button mushrooms, finely chopped

½ cup chopped yellow or red onion

2 garlic cloves, minced

1 (15-ounce) can red kidney beans, drained and rinsed

1 teaspoon smoked paprika

½ teaspoon chili powder

¼ teaspoon ground cumin

¼ teaspoon garlic powder

¼ teaspoon salt

¼ teaspoon freshly ground black pepper

2 tablespoons chopped fresh cilantro

8 (6-inch) whole-wheat or corn tortillas

Mashed avocado, for serving (optional)

Salsa or pico de gallo, for serving (optional)

Shredded lettuce, for serving (optional)

Sour cream or plain Greek yogurt, for serving (optional)

1. In a large sauté pan, heat the olive oil over medium heat. Sauté the mushrooms, onion, and garlic for 5 to 8 minutes, or until the mushrooms brown. If necessary, sauté the mushrooms in batches. Drain any excess liquid that accumulates in the pan while sautéing.

2. Add the beans, smoked paprika, chili powder, cumin, garlic powder, salt, and pepper to the pan. Sauté for 1 to 2 minutes, until aromatic.

3. Turn off the heat and mix in the cilantro. Divide the taco mixture among the tortillas. If using, top with avocado, salsa, lettuce, and sour cream as desired to serve.

Variation Tip: White button mushrooms are easy to find and most affordable when it comes to fungi, but any variety will work in these tacos. Try a variety pack with shiitake, portobello, maitake, and button mushrooms for added flavor and texture.

PER SERVING: CALORIES: 231; TOTAL FAT: 4G; SATURATED FAT: 1G; CARBOHYDRATES: 42G; FIBER: 9G; PROTEIN: 11G; SODIUM: 179MG

LENTIL SLOPPY JOES WITH TANGY CABBAGE SLAW

SERVES
4

PREP TIME:
15 minutes

COOK TIME:
50 minutes

DAIRY-FREE

VEGETARIAN

Transform a favorite childhood dinner into a lean, plant-based meal by substituting lentils for meat. Lentils are rich in iron, protein, and fiber. While the ingredient list may appear long, you likely have many ingredients in your pantry already. Using precooked lentils saves time in the cooking process and, if you want to reduce added sugar, eliminate the brown sugar or use ketchup without added sugar.

FOR THE LENTIL SLOPPY JOES

1 tablespoon extra-virgin olive oil

½ cup finely chopped yellow onion

1 green bell pepper, finely chopped

2 garlic cloves, minced

1 cup ketchup

1 tablespoon brown sugar

2 teaspoons Worcestershire sauce

2 teaspoons Dijon mustard

½ teaspoon garlic powder

¼ teaspoon smoked paprika

1½ teaspoons salt

¼ teaspoon freshly ground black pepper

2 cups cooked green lentils

4 whole-wheat hamburger buns

FOR THE CABBAGE SLAW

¼ cup red wine vinegar

3 tablespoons extra-virgin olive oil

2 tablespoons apple cider vinegar

1½ teaspoons agave syrup or honey

⅛ teaspoon salt

⅛ teaspoon freshly ground black pepper

5 cups shredded red cabbage

¼ cup thinly sliced red onion

1 thinly sliced jalapeño

2 tablespoons finely chopped fresh cilantro

TO MAKE THE LENTIL SLOPPY JOES

1. In a cast iron skillet or sauté pan, heat the olive oil over medium heat and sauté the onion and green pepper for about 5 minutes, until soft. Add the garlic and cook for about 1 minute, until fragrant.

2. Add the ketchup, 1 cup of water, brown sugar, Worcestershire, Dijon, garlic powder, smoked paprika, salt, and pepper to the skillet. Bring to a boil, then reduce to a simmer.

3. Add the cooked lentils and simmer for 25 to 30 minutes to thicken.

TO MAKE THE CABBAGE SLAW

1. While the sauce simmers, in a large bowl, mix the red wine vinegar, olive oil, apple cider vinegar, agave syrup, salt, and pepper. Add the cabbage, onion, jalapeño, and cilantro. Toss together until the cabbage is coated in dressing. Set aside.

2. Once the sauce has thickened, serve the lentil sloppy joes on hamburger buns with the cabbage slaw.

Leftovers Tip: Believe it or not, leftovers taste even better! Switch things up by changing the vehicle on which you serve these sloppy joes—try baked potatoes or any whole-grain. You can also freeze leftovers to reheat at a later date. The lentil–sloppy joe mixture will keep well in an airtight, freezer-safe container for up to 3 months.

PER SERVING: CALORIES: 455; TOTAL FAT: 17G; SATURATED FAT: 2G; CARBOHYDRATES: 68G; FIBER: 14G; PROTEIN: 15G; SODIUM: 1446MG

LENTIL "MEATBALLS" AND SPAGHETTI

SERVES
4 to 6
(1 serving =
4 pieces)

PREP TIME:
15 minutes

COOK TIME:
75 minutes

HEART HEALTHY

VEGETARIAN

Lentil "meatballs" are a great option to replace a traditional family favorite with less saturated fat and more plant-based protein and fiber. While this recipe may be more labor intensive than some others, you can prepare this recipe in stages (like making the lentils in advance) or take a shortcut, like using packaged steamed lentils you can find in the produce department. Serve over whole-wheat spaghetti, zoodles, carrot noodles, or my personal favorite, spaghetti squash.

2 cups low-sodium
  vegetable broth

1 cup green lentils

¼ cup chopped yellow onion

¼ cup grated Parmesan cheese

2 garlic cloves, peeled

2 tablespoons dried parsley

1 tablespoon tomato paste

1 tablespoon dried oregano

1 tablespoon dried basil

¼ teaspoon salt

¼ teaspoon freshly ground
  black pepper

1 large egg

1 tablespoon extra-virgin olive oil

8 ounces whole-wheat spaghetti,
  cooked, for serving

1 (28-ounce) jar marinara sauce,
  for serving

1. In a saucepan, combine the vegetable broth and lentils. Bring to a boil, then reduce to a simmer and cook for 40 to 45 minutes, or until lentils are soft and cooked. Remove from heat and let the lentils cool.

2. In a food processor, combine 2 cups of cooked lentils with the onion, Parmesan cheese, garlic, parsley, tomato paste, oregano, basil, salt, and pepper. Pulse until combined, but not fully puréed. If you do not have a food processor, you can mash the lentils well when warm with a potato masher or a fork.

3. Transfer the mixture to a bowl. Mix in the egg.

4. Preheat the oven to 375°F. Line a sheet pan with parchment paper and set aside.

5. Heat a large cast iron skillet over medium heat. When the skillet is hot, add the olive oil to the pan. Scoop a heaping tablespoon of the lentil mixture and roll into a ball. Repeat until all the lentil mixture is used. Add the lentil meatballs to the hot skillet. Cook until crispy on the outside, gently moving the balls around the skillet until browned on all sides, about 5 minutes.

6. Lentil meatballs will be delicate, so carefully transfer the balls to the prepared sheet pan and bake for 15 minutes.

7. Serve with whole-wheat spaghetti and your favorite jarred sauce.

Leftovers Tip: Leftovers will freeze great for up to 3 months. Wrap lentil balls in plastic wrap and put them in a freezer-safe bag or container.

PER SERVING: CALORIES: 506; TOTAL FAT: 8G; SATURATED FAT: 2G; CARBOHYDRATES: 86G; FIBER: 19G; PROTEIN: 29G; SODIUM: 1218MG

SHEET PAN MISO HONEY TEMPEH AND BROCCOLI

SERVES
4

PREP TIME:
10 minutes

COOK TIME:
20 minutes

30 MINUTES

DAIRY-FREE

GLUTEN-FREE

GF

HEART HEALTHY

VEGETARIAN

Nurture a healthy gut microbiome with this sheet-pan meal loaded with fermented foods. Both miso and tempeh are made from fermented soybeans, which help boost the beneficial bacteria in your gut. Enjoy this simple meal on its own or over rice.

2 tablespoons white miso paste

2 tablespoons low-sodium soy sauce

2 tablespoons avocado oil

Juice from ½ lime

1 tablespoon honey

1 teaspoon hot chili sauce

½ teaspoon finely minced peeled ginger

1 (8-ounce) package tempeh, cut into strips

6 cups broccoli florets (about 1 large head)

1. Preheat the oven to 400°F.

2. In a large bowl, mix together the miso paste, soy sauce, avocado oil, lime juice, honey, chili sauce, and ginger.

3. Add the tempeh and broccoli to the sauce and toss together.

4. Transfer the tempeh and broccoli to a large sheet pan in a single layer. Bake for 10 minutes. Remove from the oven and flip tempeh and toss the broccoli with a spatula. Return to the oven for another 10 minutes. Serve with rice or another whole-grain.

Leftovers Tip: Leftovers will make a delicious lunch tomorrow, but you may need to add more oomph to the meal. Cook a bag of frozen stir-fry vegetables and mix it into the leftovers. Add an extra splash of soy sauce, if needed.

PER SERVING: CALORIES: 254; TOTAL FAT: 14G; SATURATED FAT: 2G; CARBOHYDRATES: 23G; FIBER: 4G; PROTEIN: 16G; SODIUM: 677MG

ROASTED RED PEPPER RIGATONI

Pasta drenched in a creamy, homemade roasted red pepper sauce is a comforting meal that's easy to make in less than 30 minutes and packed with nutrients like vitamin C, folate, and antioxidants. Save time by using jarred roasted red peppers packed in water.

SERVES
4

PREP TIME:
10 minutes

COOK TIME:
15 minutes

30 MINUTES

DAIRY-FREE

HEART HEALTHY

VEGETARIAN

1 tablespoon salt, plus ¼ teaspoon

8 ounces rigatoni, penne, or gemelli pasta

1 tablespoon extra-virgin olive oil

¼ cup chopped white or yellow onion

4 jarred roasted red peppers packed in water, drained

½ teaspoon finely chopped garlic

¼ teaspoon freshly ground black pepper

¼ cup roughly chopped fresh parsley

1. In a large pot, bring 4 quarts of water and 1 tablespoon of salt to a boil. Once boiling, add the pasta and cook according to package, until al dente.

2. While the pasta cooks, in a small skillet, warm the olive oil over medium heat. Sauté the onion for about 5 minutes, until soft.

3. Transfer the onion to a blender with the roasted peppers, garlic, remaining ¼ teaspoon of salt, and pepper. Blend until smooth.

4. When the pasta is cooked, drain, reserving ¼ cup of the cooking water. Add the sauce to the pasta along with the starchy cooking water and mix together. Garnish with parsley before serving.

Substitution Tip: Boost the protein and fiber content by using lentil, chickpea, or another legume-based pasta. Many of these pasta alternatives have similar texture to pasta, but more protein and fiber (up to 11 grams of protein and 7 grams of fiber per 2 ounce serving).

PER SERVING: CALORIES: 269; TOTAL FAT: 4G; SATURATED FAT: 1G; CARBOHYDRATES: 46G; FIBER: 1G; PROTEIN: 8G; SODIUM: 430MG

MARINATED TOFU GREEK SALAD

SERVES
4

PREP TIME:
15 minutes,
plus 1 hour
to press tofu
and 1 hour to
marinate

DAIRY-FREE

GLUTEN-FREE

GF

HEART HEALTHY

VEGETARIAN

Tofu can be an intimidating ingredient to work with; however, once you make this recipe you'll see how simple it truly is! The key to working with tofu is to press out excess liquid because tofu is like a sponge and will soak up any flavor you pair it with. For this Greek salad, the dairy-free, marinated tofu mimics the flavor of tangy feta cheese thanks to miso paste, lemon juice, vinegar, nutritional yeast, and spices. You can find miso in the refrigerated section of the supermarket.

FOR THE MARINATED TOFU

1 (14-ounce) block organic extra firm tofu

2 tablespoons extra-virgin olive oil

1 tablespoon white miso paste

1 tablespoon freshly squeezed lemon juice

1 tablespoon red wine vinegar

2 tablespoons chopped fresh dill

1 tablespoon nutritional yeast

½ teaspoon dried oregano

¼ teaspoon garlic powder

⅛ teaspoon freshly ground black pepper

⅛ teaspoon sea salt

FOR THE SALAD

2 cups grape tomatoes, halved

1 cup cucumbers, cut into half moons

1 red, yellow, or orange bell pepper, chopped

¼ cup sliced pepperoncini

¼ cup chopped fresh dill

1 tablespoon extra-virgin olive oil

1. Press the tofu to remove excess moisture. If you do not own a tofu press, wrap the tofu in paper towels and set in a shallow bowl. Place a heavy-bottomed pan on top. Let sit for at least 1 hour. Once the tofu is pressed, cut into ½-inch cubes and put in a medium bowl.

2. In a small bowl, mix the olive oil, miso, lemon juice, and vinegar until emulsified and well combined. Add in the dill, nutritional yeast, oregano, garlic powder, pepper, and salt. Continue mixing until combined.

3. Pour the marinade over the tofu and gently toss until tofu is completely coated. Cover the bowl and refrigerate for at least 1 hour or as long as overnight.

TO MAKE THE SALAD

1. In a large bowl, toss the tomatoes, cucumbers, bell pepper, pepperoncini, dill, and olive oil.

2. Top with marinated tofu. Gently toss together before serving.

Leftovers Tip: Leftovers store well in the refrigerator in an airtight container for 3 to 4 days. To save time, prep this recipe in advance. Use on a sandwich, in a wrap, or even spread instead of the goat cheese on the Shredded Brussels Sprouts and Goat Cheese Flatbread (page 94).

PER SERVING: CALORIES: 293; TOTAL FAT: 21G; SATURATED FAT: 3G; CARBOHYDRATES: 12G; FIBER: 4G; PROTEIN: 18G; SODIUM: 247MG

GREEK HUMMUS COLLARD WRAPS

SERVES
4

PREP TIME:
10 minutes

30 MINUTES

GLUTEN-FREE

GF

HEART HEALTHY

VEGETARIAN

Collard wraps are a fun, low-carb way to eat more veggies. By using vegetables instead of bread, you'll enjoy more antioxidants, vitamins, and minerals with every delicious bite. Rolling a collard wrap takes a bit of practice, but it's similar to rolling a burrito. If you have trouble with raw collard leaves, you can steam the leaves for a few minutes to soften them.

8 to 10 large collard leaves
1 cup hummus
½ cup crumbled feta cheese
½ cup thinly sliced cucumber
1 large tomato, sliced

2 cups alfalfa or broccoli sprouts
½ cup sliced red onion
¼ teaspoon sumac
¼ teaspoon dried oregano

1. Separate the collards and carefully shave down the spine on the back of each leaf using a small, sharp knife.

2. Spread about 2 tablespoons of hummus on each leaf, then top with 1 tablespoon of crumbled feta cheese, followed by cucumber, tomato, sprouts, onions, sumac, and oregano to your liking.

3. To form each wrap, fold in the top and bottom of the leaf, then roll it up. Place seam-side down on your plate to stay secure.

Substitution Tip: Looking for more oomph in your wrap? Bulk up your meal by making half of your wraps using a high-fiber whole-wheat wrap instead of collard greens.

PER SERVING: CALORIES: 195; TOTAL FAT: 11G; SATURATED FAT: 4G; CARBOHYDRATES: 18G; FIBER: 8G; PROTEIN: 11G; SODIUM: 465MG

BLACK BEAN AND MANGO SALAD STUFFED AVOCADOS

Hearty black beans pair well with sweet mango for a meat-free meal that will please your taste buds and provide a boost of protein and fiber. The recipe calls for canned black beans to save time, but you can prepare your own black beans using dried beans.

SERVES
4

PREP TIME:
15 minutes

30 MINUTES

DAIRY-FREE

GLUTEN-FREE
GF

HEART HEALTHY

VEGETARIAN

2 avocados, halved lengthwise

½ teaspoon salt, divided

1 (15-ounce) can low-sodium black beans, drained and rinsed

1 mango, chopped

¼ cup plus 2 tablespoons chopped red onion

¼ cup finely chopped yellow bell pepper

¼ cup chopped fresh cilantro

Juice from 1 lime

⅛ teaspoon freshly ground black pepper

1. Place the avocado halves on a plate. Sprinkle with ¼ teaspoon of salt and set aside.

2. In a large bowl, toss the black beans, mango, red onion, bell pepper, cilantro, lime juice, ¼ teaspoon of salt, and pepper.

3. Spoon the bean and mango salad over the avocados.

Substitution Tip: If avocados are out of season or experiencing a spike in price, use another edible vehicle to contain the black bean and mango salad. Try roasted sweet potatoes, butternut squash, or a scooped-out tomato.

PER SERVING: CALORIES: 245; TOTAL FAT: 14G; SATURATED FAT: 2G; CARBOHYDRATES: 30G; FIBER: 11G; PROTEIN: 6G; SODIUM: 359MG

TOTALLY LOADED SWEET POTATO NACHOS

SERVES
4

PREP TIME:
10 minutes

COOK TIME:
35 minutes

GLUTEN-FREE
GF

VEGETARIAN

Nachos get a healthy makeover by swapping nutrient-dense sweet potatoes for tortilla chips. Be sure not to overcrowd your sheet pan in order to get crispy sweet potato rounds. Topped with melted cheddar cheese, black beans, salsa, avocado, scallions, jalapeño, and cilantro, this is a weeknight meal your entire family will love! Plus, this is a great recipe to entertain with as you can double or triple the recipe when feeding a crowd.

4 medium sweet potatoes or yams, cut into ⅛-inch slices

1 tablespoon avocado oil

¼ teaspoon salt

1 (15-ounce) can low-sodium black beans, drained and rinsed

1 cup shredded cheddar cheese or Mexican blend cheese

½ cup jarred or fresh salsa

1 avocado, sliced

¼ cup sliced scallions, green part only

1 jalapeño, sliced (optional)

2 tablespoons chopped fresh cilantro

1. Preheat the oven to 400°F.

2. In a large bowl, toss the sweet potato slices in avocado oil to coat. Distribute on a sheet pan in a single layer and sprinkle with salt. If necessary, roast the sweet potatoes on two sheet pans.

3. Roast for 15 minutes. Using a spatula, flip the potato slices and return to oven to roast for another 10 to 15 minutes, until cooked through and crispy at the edges.

4. Move the slices close together on the sheet pan and top with the beans and cheese. Return to the oven for another 5 minutes, until the cheese melts.

5. Remove the nachos from the oven and top with salsa, avocado slices, scallions, jalapeño slices (if using), and cilantro. Dig in!

Variation Tip: Set up a "nacho bar" for a fun weeknight dinner with your kids. After the sweet potato rounds cook and the cheese melts, divide among individual plates. Add several toppings to bowls and let your family top their own sweet potato nachos.

PER SERVING: CALORIES: 381; TOTAL FAT: 20G; SATURATED FAT: 7G; CARBOHYDRATES: 40G; FIBER: 11G; PROTEIN: 14G; SODIUM: 653MG

SHREDDED BRUSSELS SPROUTS AND GOAT CHEESE FLATBREAD

SERVES
4

PREP TIME:
15 minutes

COOK TIME:
20 minutes

VEGETARIAN

The antioxidants and phytonutrients in Brussels sprouts promote incredible health benefits, including DNA protection, cancer prevention, cholesterol-lowering effects, and more. In fact, Brussels sprouts are thought to be one of the healthiest cruciferous vegetables. Save time preparing this recipe by using store-bought shredded sprouts. If you can't find whole-wheat naan in your supermarket, opt for whole-wheat pita bread to boost your intake of whole-grains and fiber.

1 tablespoon extra-virgin olive oil

2 cups thinly sliced red onion

6 cups shredded Brussels sprouts

¼ teaspoon garlic powder

⅛ teaspoon salt

⅛ teaspoon freshly ground
black pepper

¼ cup dried cranberries

4 pieces whole-wheat naan

4 ounces goat cheese, at room
temperature

2 tablespoons grated
Parmesan cheese

1. Preheat the oven to 400°F.

2. In a large sauté pan, heat the olive oil over low to medium heat. Sauté the onion for about 5 minutes, until softened.

3. Add the shredded Brussels sprouts, garlic powder, salt, and pepper, continuing to sauté for another 3 minutes until soft. Mix in the dried cranberries. Set aside.

4. Place the naan on a large sheet pan. Spread the goat cheese on top.

5. Distribute the Brussels sprouts mixture on top of the goat cheese. Sprinkle ½ tablespoon Parmesan cheese on top of each flatbread.

6. Bake the flatbreads for 10 minutes, until the edges are crispy. Enjoy warm.

Substitution Tip: There are many simple swaps you can make for this recipe, depending on what you have available in your pantry. Try ricotta cheese instead of goat cheese, shredded kale instead of Brussels sprouts (you may need to reduce the cooking time), or raisins or chopped dates instead of dried cranberries.

PER SERVING: CALORIES: 390; TOTAL FAT: 12G; SATURATED FAT: 6G; CARBOHYDRATES: 59G; FIBER: 11G; PROTEIN: 18G; SODIUM: 586MG

WHOLE ROASTED CAULIFLOWER WITH SUNFLOWER SEED PESTO

SERVES
4

PREP TIME:
10 minutes

COOK TIME:
1 hour 18 minutes

DAIRY-FREE

GLUTEN-FREE
GF

HEART HEALTHY

VEGETARIAN

Did you know you can roast a head of cauliflower whole for a tender-on-the-inside, crispy-on-the-outside vegetable? This dish is simple to prepare with largely hands-off roasting time, so you can set it and (almost) forget it. Impress guests with this healthy dish, perfect as a main course or a scrumptious side.

FOR THE WHOLE ROASTED CAULIFLOWER

1 large head cauliflower, stem and leaves removed

1 tablespoon avocado oil

¼ teaspoon smoked paprika

¼ teaspoon salt

⅛ teaspoon freshly ground black pepper

⅛ teaspoon garlic powder

¼ teaspoon dried parsley

FOR THE SUNFLOWER SEED PESTO

3 cups fresh basil

¼ cup sunflower seeds

¼ cup extra-virgin olive oil

2 garlic cloves, peeled

Zest from 1 medium lemon

1 teaspoon freshly squeezed lemon juice

½ teaspoon sea salt

TO MAKE THE WHOLE ROASTED CAULIFLOWER

1. Preheat the oven to 425°F.

2. Place the cauliflower in an 8-by-8-inch baking dish. If the cauliflower will not lay flat, cut the bottom of the cauliflower to create a flat surface.

3. Coat the head of cauliflower with avocado oil, then sprinkle with smoked paprika, salt, pepper, garlic powder, and dried parsley.

4. Cover with aluminum foil and roast for 1 hour and 15 minutes, or until fork-tender. Remove the foil and set the broiler to high. Broil for 3 minutes, until the top of the cauliflower is crispy.

TO MAKE THE SUNFLOWER SEED PESTO

1. While the cauliflower is roasting, in a food processor, combine the basil, sunflower seeds, olive oil, garlic, lemon zest, lemon juice, and salt. Process until smooth. You may need to pause to scrape down the sides of the food processor. To thin the pesto more, add additional oil.

2. To assemble, drizzle the pesto on top of the cauliflower. Cut the head into large slices for a "steak"-like presentation. Garnish with fresh basil and sunflower seeds, if desired.

Leftovers Tip: Chop up leftover cauliflower and add to a salad for tomorrow's lunch. The pesto acts as a delicious dressing, too! Leftover pesto can also be used on top of pasta or fish for a quick dinner tomorrow night.

PER SERVING: CALORIES: 226; TOTAL FAT: 19G; SATURATED FAT: 3G; CARBOHYDRATES: 13G; FIBER: 6G; PROTEIN: 6G; SODIUM: 503MG

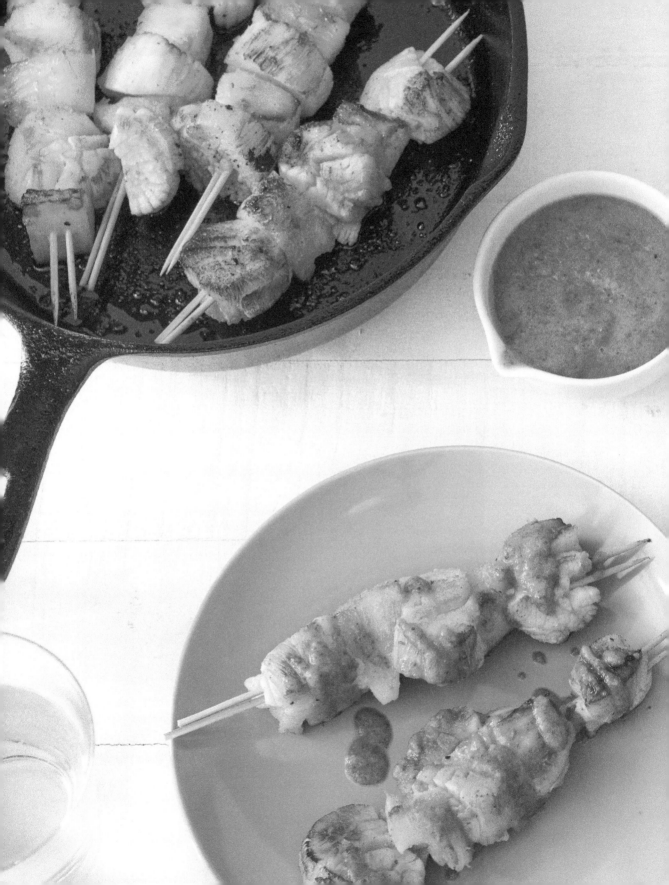

CHAPTER SEVEN

FISH AND SEAFOOD MAINS

SHEET PAN JERK FISH TACOS

SERVES
4

PREP TIME:
10 minutes

COOK TIME:
10 minutes

30 MINUTES

DAIRY-FREE

HEART HEALTHY

Jamaican jerk seasoning adds a punch of heat and a pinch of sweetness to taco night. Using a rub with a variety of spices is a great way to enhance the flavor of your meal without adding many calories or fat. Don't underestimate the value of a well-stocked spice cabinet for flavor and health benefits! You can double or triple the seasoning and store in an airtight container for future use, too!

FOR THE JAMAICAN JERK SEASONING

2 teaspoons garlic powder

2 teaspoons onion powder

2 teaspoons dried parsley

2 teaspoons dried thyme

2 teaspoons light brown sugar

1 teaspoon smoked paprika

1 teaspoon red pepper flakes

1 teaspoon salt

½ teaspoon freshly ground
   black pepper

½ teaspoon ground allspice

¼ teaspoon ground cinnamon

FOR THE FISH TACOS

4 (6-ounce) flounder fillets

2 cups sliced yellow onion

1 teaspoon avocado oil

8 corn or whole-wheat tortillas

¼ cup roughly chopped fresh
   cilantro

Juice from ½ lime

In a small bowl, combine the garlic powder, onion powder, parsley, thyme, brown sugar, paprika, red pepper flakes, salt, pepper, allspice, and cinnamon.

TO MAKE THE FISH TACOS

1. Preheat the oven to 375°F. Line a sheet pan with parchment paper.

2. Place the flounder fillets on the prepared sheet pan. Sprinkle about 1 tablespoon of the seasoning on top of each of the fish fillets. The fish should be completely covered with the seasoning.

3. Toss the onion slices in avocado oil and 2 teaspoons of the jerk seasoning. Place on the sheet pan next to the fish.

4. Bake the fish and onions for 10 minutes, or until the fish flakes with a fork.

5. While the fish bakes, in a dry skillet, heat the tortillas over medium-high heat until warm.

6. To assemble the tacos, divide the fish and onions among the tortillas. Top with cilantro and a squeeze of lime.

Substitution Tip: This recipe works well for any white, flaky fish, including snapper, tilapia, sole, and more. For a low-carb alternative, use butter lettuce or romaine lettuce leaves instead of tortillas.

PER SERVING: CALORIES: 421; TOTAL FAT: 12G; SATURATED FAT: 1G; CARBOHYDRATES: 41G; FIBER: 4G; PROTEIN: 38G; SODIUM: 1125MG

PEPITA PESTO-CRUSTED COD

SERVES
4

PREP TIME:
5 minutes

COOK TIME:
25 to 27
minutes

30 MINUTES

DAIRY-FREE

HEART HEALTHY

Elevate plain fish with a tasty pesto topping that combines the earthy flavor of pumpkin seeds with spicy arugula and sweet basil. Toasting the pepitas adds depth to their flavor, so don't skip this step! Prepare the pesto in advance for a quick meal and you can make in less than 30 minutes. If cod is not available, use this pepita pesto on any flaky white fish, like halibut, snapper, sole, or tilapia.

FOR THE PEPITA PESTO

½ cup pepitas

4 cups fresh basil

2 cups arugula

⅓ cup extra-virgin olive oil

3 garlic cloves, peeled

¾ teaspoon sea salt

¼ cup whole-wheat
  bread crumbs

FOR THE COD

4 (6-ounce) cod fillets, about
  1-inch thick

Salt

Freshly ground black pepper

1. Heat a small skillet over medium heat. Toast the pepitas for 5 to 7 minutes, constantly moving them around the pan to prevent burning.

2. Add the toasted pepitas, basil, arugula, olive oil, garlic, and salt to a food processor. Pulse until combined. Mix in the bread crumbs.

1. Preheat the oven to 350°F. Line a large sheet pan with parchment paper.

2. Place the fish on the sheet pan. Sprinkle with salt and pepper. Divide the pesto among the cod fillets and spread in an even layer.

3. Bake for 15 to 20 minutes, until the fish is opaque and the flesh flakes easily with a fork.

Leftovers Tip: Repurpose leftover pesto on pasta with shrimp the following night. Pan-sear shrimp and prepare the pasta according to package. Toss together with pesto and enjoy!

PER SERVING: CALORIES: 397; TOTAL FAT: 26G; SATURATED FAT: 4G; CARBOHYDRATES: 9G; FIBER: 1G; PROTEIN: 36G; SODIUM: 551MG

SLOW-ROASTED DIJON ARCTIC CHAR

SERVES
4

PREP TIME:
10 minutes

COOK TIME:
20 minutes

30 MINUTES

DAIRY-FREE

GLUTEN-FREE

GF

HEART HEALTHY

This is the recipe I keep in my back pocket for when I'm in a rush to make dinner and don't know what to do with a piece of fish. Although the recipe says "slow-roasted," the fish cooks so quickly that you can prepare this recipe in under 30 minutes. Turning down the oven temperature and layering Dijon mustard on top of a beautiful fillet ensures the fish doesn't dry out.

4 (6-ounce) arctic char fillets
1 teaspoon smoked paprika
¼ teaspoon salt
¼ teaspoon freshly ground
   black pepper

¼ cup Dijon mustard
1 teaspoon light or dark
   brown sugar

1. Preheat the oven to 300°F.

2. Place the arctic char fillets on a sheet pan. Season with smoked paprika, salt, and pepper. Spread the mustard on top of the fish. Sprinkle the brown sugar on top.

3. Bake the fish for 20 minutes, until it flakes easily with a fork.

Substitution Tip: Arctic char not available or in season? Use salmon instead. Both fish have pink flesh with a flaky outcome.

PER SERVING: CALORIES: 321; TOTAL FAT: 4G; SATURATED FAT: 2G; CARBOHYDRATES: 2G; FIBER: 1G; PROTEIN: 37G; SODIUM: 358MG

SHEET PAN "LOW COUNTRY SHRIMP BOIL"

Sheet pan meals are an easy way to serve a healthy dinner with minimal clean up. This sheet pan shrimp dinner is inspired by a "low country boil," which traditionally combines red potatoes, corn, and seafood, plus seafood's favorite seasoning—Old Bay. Serve with a side salad to add some greens to your plate.

SERVES
6

PREP TIME:
15 minutes

COOK TIME:
27 minutes

DAIRY-FREE

GLUTEN-FREE
GF

1 ½ pounds red potatoes, quartered

2 large yellow onions, quartered

2 corn ears, cut into ½-inch pieces

2 tablespoons extra-virgin olive oil, divided

4 teaspoons Old Bay Seasoning, divided

1 ½ pounds 21/25 count shrimp, peeled and deveined

1. Preheat the oven to 400°F.

2. In a large bowl, toss the potatoes, onions, corn, 1½ tablespoons of olive oil, and 2½ teaspoons of Old Bay.

3. Transfer to a large sheet pan and roast for 20 minutes. Do not overcrowd the sheet pan. If needed, use two sheet pans.

4. While the vegetables roast, rinse the shrimp and pat dry. In the same bowl, toss the shrimp in in the remaining ½ tablespoon of oil and 1½ teaspoons of Old Bay.

5. After 20 minutes, remove the sheet pan from the oven. Switch the oven to broil. Add the shrimp to the sheet pan. Broil for 7 minutes, until the shrimp are opaque and cooked through.

Variation Tip: If fresh corn is not in season, use frozen and thawed corn on the cob or kernels. If using frozen corn kernels, add them to the sheet pan when you broil the shrimp.

PER SERVING: CALORIES: 318; TOTAL FAT: 7G; SATURATED FAT: 1G; CARBOHYDRATES: 34G; FIBER: 4G; PROTEIN: 30G; SODIUM: 720MG

NO-FUSS CRAB CAKES WITH TZATZIKI SAUCE

SERVES
4

PREP TIME:
15 minutes

30 MINUTES

These no-fuss crab cakes really are no fuss! They're made in one bowl and in less than 30 minutes from start to finish! Unlike typical crab cakes, this recipe uses whole-wheat bread crumbs to bump up the fiber and nutrients and is paired with a tzatziki sauce instead of tartar sauce.

FOR THE TZATZIKI SAUCE

1 cup plain low-fat Greek yogurt

½ cup shredded cucumber

¼ cup chopped fresh dill

1 tablespoon extra-virgin olive oil

1 tablespoon freshly squeezed lemon juice

1 garlic clove, minced

⅛ teaspoon salt

⅛ teaspoon ground white pepper

FOR THE CRAB CAKES

8 ounces jumbo lump crabmeat, picked over to remove remaining shell pieces

½ cup whole-wheat panko bread crumbs

1 large egg

2 scallions, both white and green parts, chopped

3 tablespoons coarsely chopped parsley

2 tablespoons Dijon mustard

2 tablespoons mayonnaise

1 teaspoon Worcestershire sauce

½ teaspoon Old Bay Seasoning

¼ teaspoon salt

¼ teaspoon freshly ground black pepper

1 tablespoon avocado oil

In a medium bowl, combine the yogurt, cucumber, dill, olive oil, lemon juice, garlic, salt, and white pepper. Cover and refrigerate while you prepare and cook the crab cakes.

FOR THE CRAB CAKES

1. In a medium bowl, mix together the crab, bread crumbs, egg, scallions, parsley, Dijon, mayonnaise, Worcestershire, Old Bay, salt, and pepper.

2. In a cast iron skillet, heat the avocado oil over medium-high heat. Using a ⅓-cup measuring cup, form the crab mixture into 6 patties, flattening them to ½-inch thick.

3. Cook for 3 to 4 minutes on each side, until a golden brown crust forms. Using a spatula, transfer them to a paper towel–lined plate. Serve with tzatziki sauce.

Variation Tip: For a crispy exterior, these crab cakes are pan-fried; however, you can bake them at 375°F for 25 to 30 minutes, flipping halfway through.

PER SERVING: CALORIES: 283; TOTAL FAT: 16G; SATURATED FAT: 2G; CARBOHYDRATES: 15G; FIBER: 2G; PROTEIN: 22G; SODIUM: 672MG

LEMON-CAPER FISH AND VEGGIES EN PAPILLOTE

SERVES
4

PREP TIME:
10 minutes

COOK TIME:
13 to 15
minutes

30 MINUTES

GLUTEN-FREE

GF

HEART HEALTHY

Cooking fish *en papillote* is a great way to dip your toes into the ocean of cooking fish. Bake fish in a parchment paper pouch to steam the contents of the pouch, creating a tender outcome that's hard to mess up! Haricot verts have similar cooking time to the fish, making them a simple pair, but you can easily substitute asparagus, mushrooms, peppers, or zucchini, too.

1 pound haricot verts

4 (6-ounce) white fish fillets (flounder, snapper, or tilapia), about ½-inch thick

½ teaspoon salt

½ teaspoon freshly ground black pepper

½ teaspoon garlic powder

4 teaspoons unsalted butter

4 teaspoons capers

1 cup chopped fresh parsley

2 lemons, thinly sliced

1. Preheat the oven to 400°F.

2. Prepare four large pieces of parchment paper that are each large enough to fold over your fish fillet, with a couple of inches of a border.

3. To assemble one packet, place one-quarter of the green beans in a single layer on the lower half of each piece of parchment paper. Place each fish fillet on top of each layer of green beans. Season each with ⅛ teaspoon of salt, pepper, and garlic powder. Top the fish with a pat of butter (about 1 teaspoon), 1 teaspoon of capers, ¼ cup of parsley, and 3 or 4 lemon slices.

4. Fold the parchment paper over the fish and fold down the edges, sealing the fish and veggies in a packet. Place on a sheet pan. Repeat with the remaining ingredients to create four packets.

5. Bake for 13 to 15 minutes, until the fish is cooked through and flakes with a fork. Cooking time varies with the thickness of the fish; adjust as necessary.

6. Remove from the oven and let sit for a couple of minutes, until cool to the touch.

7. Carefully open the parchment paper packets, allowing the steam to escape.

Substitution Tip: This recipe calls for a mild white fish; however, you can use any fish and an assortment of vegetables using this cooking method. Adjust the cooking time based on the thickness of your fish.

PER SERVING: CALORIES: 208; TOTAL FAT: 6G; SATURATED FAT: 3G; CARBOHYDRATES: 8G; FIBER: 5G; PROTEIN: 34G; SODIUM: 471MG

GRILLED SCALLOP AND PINEAPPLE SKEWERS WITH ROASTED POBLANO PEPPER SAUCE

SERVES
4

PREP TIME:
20 minutes,
plus 30 minutes
for soaking
wooden
skewers

COOK TIME:
18 minutes

DAIRY-FREE

GLUTEN-FREE

GF

HEART HEALTHY

Mildly spicy poblano peppers are roasted to reveal a sweeter flavor, then blended together with fresh cilantro and lime juice for a sauce that pops on grilled scallops and pineapple. This is the perfect summer recipe to entertain with, especially paired with the Shaved Fennel, Corn, and Peach Salad (page 60). Be sure to soak wooden skewers in water for 30 minutes before threading to prevent scorching.

FOR THE ROASTED POBLANO PEPPER SAUCE

2 poblano peppers

½ cup freshly squeezed lime juice

½ cup finely chopped fresh cilantro

2 tablespoons extra-virgin olive oil

2 tablespoons agave syrup

¼ teaspoon salt

⅛ teaspoon freshly ground black pepper

FOR THE SKEWERS

1 pound scallops

2 cups chopped pineapple, cut into 2-inch pieces

1 tablespoon avocado oil

Juice from ½ lime

½ teaspoon garlic powder

½ teaspoon smoked paprika

½ teaspoon chili powder

¼ teaspoon salt

¼ teaspoon freshly ground black pepper

TO MAKE THE ROASTED POBLANO PEPPER SAUCE

1. Preheat the oven to broil. Place the peppers on a sheet pan and broil for 10 minutes, turning every 2 to 3 minutes with tongs. The peppers should be well done, with the skin charred and easy to remove when done. Once peppers cool to the touch, remove the skin and seeds from the peppers.

2. In a blender, combine the poblano pepper flesh, lime juice, cilantro, olive oil, agave syrup, salt, and pepper. Process until smooth. Transfer to a small bowl and set aside.

TO MAKE THE SKEWERS

1. Pat the scallops dry.

2. In a large bowl, toss the scallops and pineapple with the avocado oil, lime juice, garlic powder, smoked paprika, chili powder, salt, and pepper.

3. Alternate threading the scallops and pineapple onto wooden skewers, using two skewers per kebob. Repeat until all scallops and pineapple are used.

4. Heat the grill to medium-high heat. Place the skewers directly over the heat on a greased grill rack for 8 minutes, flipping halfway through, until the scallops are opaque.

5. Drizzle the roasted poblano pepper sauce on top before serving.

Variation Tip: To prepare this recipe indoors, cook the scallops and pineapple in a cast iron pan. Heat 1 tablespoon of oil in the pan over high heat. Add the skewers and cook for 8 minutes, rotating halfway through, until scallops are opaque.

PER SERVING: CALORIES: 285; TOTAL FAT: 12G; SATURATED FAT: 2G; CARBOHYDRATES: 28G; FIBER: 2G; PROTEIN: 20G; SODIUM: 488MG

MASON JAR SUSHI SALAD

SERVES
4

PREP TIME:
15 minutes

COOK TIME:
45 minutes

DAIRY-FREE

HEART HEALTHY

Enjoy sushi at home without the hassle of learning how to craft the perfect sushi roll. With a combination of carbohydrates, lean protein, and healthy fats, this sushi salad puts the best aspects of a sushi bar into one jar! Adding the dressing to the bottom of the jar keeps the salad contents from getting soggy. Prep these jars in advance for a quick lunch to take on the go.

FOR THE GINGER DRESSING

½ cup finely chopped yellow onion

¼ cup shredded carrots

¼ cup rice vinegar

2½ tablespoons finely minced peeled ginger

1½ tablespoons honey

1 tablespoon low-sodium soy sauce

1 teaspoon hot chili sauce

½ teaspoon minced garlic

FOR THE SUSHI SALAD

1 cup short-grain brown rice

1 cup shelled edamame, fresh or frozen and thawed

1 cup julienned cucumber

1 cup shredded carrots

6 ounces crabmeat or your favorite sushi-grade fish

2 seaweed sheets, crumbled or cut into thin strips

In a high-powered blender or food processor, combine the onion, carrots, rice vinegar, ginger, honey, soy sauce, chili sauce, garlic, and 2 tablespoons of water. Blend until mostly smooth.

TO MAKE THE SUSHI SALAD

1. In a medium saucepan, combine 2 cups of water and the rice. Bring to a boil, then reduce the heat to low, cover, and simmer for 45 minutes. Allow rice to cool slightly before assembling jars.

2. Divide the dressing among four mason jars. Layer in the rice, edamame, cucumber, carrots, and crabmeat. Garnish with shredded seaweed. Shake jars before eating.

Substitution Tip: To save time on prep work, use a store-bought ginger dressing or simply soy sauce.

Variation Tip: Make these salads gluten-free by using coconut aminos instead of soy sauce.

PER SERVING: CALORIES: 278; TOTAL FAT: 2G; SATURATED FAT: 0G; CARBOHYDRATES: 50G; FIBER: 4G; PROTEIN: 10G; SODIUM: 548MG

BRUSCHETTA BRANZINO

SERVES
4

PREP TIME:
10 minutes

COOK TIME:
8 minutes

30 MINUTES

DAIRY-FREE

GLUTEN-FREE

GF

HEART HEALTHY

Branzino is Mediterranean sea bass, a simple white fish that pairs well with flavors of the Mediterranean, like fresh tomato bruschetta. Prepare the bruschetta topping first to allow the flavors to marinate together while you prepare the fish. This dish is light, fresh, and elegant, but easy to prepare.

FOR THE BRUSCHETTA

1 cup chopped cherry or grape tomatoes

½ cup fresh basil chiffonade

2 tablespoons finely chopped red onion

1 garlic clove, finely chopped

⅛ teaspoon sea salt

FOR THE BRANZINO

1 tablespoon extra-virgin olive oil, divided

4 (6-ounce) Branzino fillets, with skin

½ teaspoon sea salt

¼ teaspoon freshly ground black pepper

In a large bowl, toss together the tomatoes, basil, red onion, garlic, and salt. Set aside.

TO MAKE THE BRANZINO

1. In a cast iron skillet, heat ½ tablespoon of the olive oil over medium-high heat.

2. Season the fish with salt and pepper on both sides.

3. Once the oil is hot, place two of the fillets, skin-side down, in the skillet. Sear for 5 minutes on the skin side before carefully flipping. Let cook for another 3 minutes, until the fish flakes with a fork. Repeat with the remaining oil and two other fillets.

4. Top the fish with bruschetta before serving.

Substitution Tip: Use any mild-flavored white fish in this recipe, such as cod, sea bream, flounder, tilapia, or sole.

PER SERVING: CALORIES: 207; TOTAL FAT: 7G; SATURATED FAT: 1G; CARBOHYDRATES: 3G; FIBER: 1G; PROTEIN: 32G; SODIUM: 349MG

HEALTHY BAKED FISH AND CHIPS

SERVES
4

PREP TIME:
15 minutes

COOK TIME:
30 minutes

DAIRY-FREE

HEART HEALTHY

As a healthier twist on classic English pub fare, even fish skeptics will love this version of fish and chips that won't leave you feeling weighed down! The secret to a delicious outcome is seasoning the fish every step of the way, including the flour, egg, and bread crumbs. Bake the "chips" and fish in the oven or use an air fryer.

2 pounds baby gold
   potatoes, halved

2 tablespoons avocado oil

½ teaspoon Old Bay
   Seasoning, divided

1 teaspoon salt, divided

4 (6-ounce) cod fillets, cut
   into strips

¼ teaspoon freshly ground black
   pepper, divided

½ cup all-purpose flour

2 large eggs

1 cup seasoned whole-wheat
   bread crumbs

1. Preheat the oven to 375°F.

2. In a large bowl, toss the potatoes in avocado oil, ¼ teaspoon of Old Bay, and ½ teaspoon of salt. Transfer to a large sheet pan. Be careful not to overcrowd the pan.

3. Roast the potatoes for 35 minutes, tossing halfway through.

4. While the potatoes are roasting, season the cod with ¼ teaspoon of salt and ⅛ teaspoon of pepper.

5. Set up a breading workspace. Pour the flour on a plate and season with the remaining ¼ teaspoon of salt. In a medium, shallow bowl, whisk the eggs with the remaining ⅛ teaspoon of pepper. Last, on a second plate, mix the bread crumbs with the remaining ¼ teaspoon of Old Bay.

6. To bread the fish, dredge in flour, then dip the fish in egg, allowing the excess to drip off. Last, coat the fish in bread crumbs. Place on a sheet pan and repeat with the remaining fish.

7. Bake for 15 minutes, flipping halfway through, until the fish flakes with a fork. Serve with the crispy potatoes.

Variation Tip: You can prepare this recipe in an air fryer, too! Follow the same steps above, except when you are ready to cook the potatoes, put them in the air fryer basket and cook on 400°F for 20 minutes, shaking the basket halfway through. Then, cook the fish on 400°F for 15 minutes, flipping halfway through. Cook in batches and do not overcrowd the air fryer basket.

PER SERVING: CALORIES: 533; TOTAL FAT: 13G; SATURATED FAT: 2G; CARBOHYDRATES: 64G; FIBER: 7G; PROTEIN: 41G; SODIUM: 980MG

CAJUN-SPICED SNAPPER WITH PINEAPPLE SALSA

SERVES
4

PREP TIME:
15 minutes

COOK TIME:
5 to 7 minutes

30 MINUTES

DAIRY-FREE

GLUTEN-FREE

GF

HEART HEALTHY

Using a spice rub is a great way to add layers of flavor to fish and health benefits, too. This Cajun seasoning contains many spice cabinet staples for a smoky and spicy kick that pairs well with the sweet pineapple salsa. Serve on its own or pair with a starchy carbohydrate, like rice or the Easy Roasted Plantains with Cilantro on page 140, for a well-balanced meal.

FOR THE CAJUN SEASONING

2 tablespoons smoked paprika

1 tablespoon sea salt

1 tablespoon garlic powder

1 tablespoon freshly ground black pepper

1 teaspoon Italian seasoning

1 teaspoon ground cayenne pepper

½ tablespoon dried thyme

FOR THE SNAPPER

4 (6-ounce) snapper fillets, about ¼- to ½-inch thick

2 cups chopped pineapple

¼ cup finely chopped red onion

¼ cup roughly chopped fresh cilantro

¼ teaspoon chili powder

In a small container or jar, combine the smoked paprika, salt, garlic powder, pepper, Italian seasoning, cayenne, and thyme. Mix well.

TO MAKE THE SNAPPER

1. Place the fish skin-side down on a large sheet pan. Generously rub about 1 tablespoon of the spice mixture on top, until the fish is completely coated. You will have leftover seasoning. Broil for 5 to 7 minutes, until the fish flakes with a fork. Cooking time may vary slightly depending on the thickness of the fish.

2. While the fish cooks, in a medium bowl, toss together the pineapple, red onion, cilantro, and chili powder.

3. When the fish is done cooking, top with pineapple salsa and serve warm.

Leftovers Tip: Store leftover Cajun seasoning in an airtight container for quick preparation the next time you make this recipe. Spices will stay fresh for up to a year.

PER SERVING: CALORIES: 294; TOTAL FAT: 4G; SATURATED FAT: 0G; CARBOHYDRATES: 17G; FIBER: 4G; PROTEIN: 46G; SODIUM: 1511MG

ORANGE-GLAZED SHRIMP STIR-FRY

SERVES
4

PREP TIME:
10 minutes

COOK TIME:
12 minutes

30 MINUTES

DAIRY-FREE

GLUTEN-FREE
GF

Shrimp is one of the quickest-cooking seafood options, making them a great weeknight protein to prepare in minutes. This quick-to-make orange glaze packs tons of flavor with minimal effort, thanks to orange marmalade. This stir-fry may be served with rice, cauliflower rice, or on its own.

3 tablespoons orange marmalade

2 tablespoons freshly squeezed orange juice

1 tablespoon low-sodium soy sauce

1 teaspoon hot chili sauce

¼ teaspoon finely chopped garlic

¼ teaspoon ground ginger

⅛ teaspoon freshly ground black pepper

1 pound shrimp, peeled and deveined

2 cups sliced white button mushrooms

2 cups sliced zucchini

2 red bell peppers, sliced

1 tablespoon avocado oil

1. In a large bowl, combine the orange marmalade, orange juice, soy sauce, chili sauce, garlic, ginger, and pepper. Transfer half of the mixture to another large bowl.

2. Put the shrimp in one bowl and the mushrooms, zucchini, and bell peppers in the other. Toss both bowls until well coated. Let sit for 5 minutes to marinate.

3. In a large sauté pan, heat the avocado oil over medium-high heat. Add the vegetables, tossing often for 5 minutes.

4. Add the shrimp to the pan. Cook for 6 to 7 minutes, until opaque. Serve over rice.

Variation Tip: Transform this recipe into a sheet pan meal by cooking the shrimp and vegetables on a large sheet pan at 400°F for 5 minutes. Then switch the oven to broil for 3 to 5 minutes, until shrimp are cooked through.

PER SERVING: CALORIES: 209; TOTAL FAT: 5G; SATURATED FAT: 0G; CARBOHYDRATES: 19G; FIBER: 2G; PROTEIN: 26G; SODIUM: 399MG

30-MINUTE MUSSELS MARINARA

Cooking mussels may seem intimidating, but they're simple and quick to prepare, especially when paired with a delicious red sauce. The key is to ensure that all shells open once cooked. Discard any mussels that do not open. You can prepare the sauce in advance, then reheat to cook the mussels just before serving.

SERVES
4

PREP TIME:
10 minutes

COOK TIME:
20 minutes

30 MINUTES

DAIRY-FREE

HEART HEALTHY

2 tablespoons extra-virgin olive oil

2 cups finely chopped yellow onion

3 garlic cloves, minced

¾ cup dry white wine, like Pinot Grigio

2 (28-ounce) cans crushed tomatoes

½ cup chopped fresh parsley

¼ cup chopped fresh basil

¾ teaspoon salt

½ teaspoon dried oregano

¼ teaspoon freshly ground black pepper

4 pounds fresh mussels, scrubbed and rinsed

8 ounces whole-wheat pasta, cooked for serving

1. In a large stock pot, heat the olive oil over medium heat. Add the onion and garlic and sauté for 2 to 3 minutes, until softened and fragrant.

2. Add the wine and bring to a boil. Then reduce the heat to a simmer and add the tomatoes, parsley, basil, salt, oregano, and pepper. Simmer for 10 minutes to reduce slightly.

3. Add the mussels to the pan and cook for 8 to 10 minutes, until all the mussels open. Discard any mussels that do not open. Serve over pasta.

Variation Tip: To amp up the heat and create a fra diavolo–style dish, add 1 to 2 teaspoons red pepper flakes while the sauce simmers.

PER SERVING: CALORIES: 415; TOTAL FAT: 11G; SATURATED FAT: 2G; CARBOHYDRATES: 45G; FIBER: 14G; PROTEIN: 29G; SODIUM: 1338MG

TUNA AVOCADO BURGERS

SERVES
4

PREP TIME:
10 minutes

COOK TIME:
20 minutes

30 MINUTES

DAIRY-FREE

HEART HEALTHY

Tuna avocado burgers are an inexpensive way to fit fish into your weekly diet, with a boost of healthy fats from avocado. To avoid green burgers, do not mash the avocado, but carefully mix instead. The patties are delicate, which is why it is best to bake them in the oven. If you wish to grill these burgers, do so on a piece of aluminum foil sprayed with nonstick spray on top of your grill.

2 (5-ounce) cans water-packed albacore tuna, drained

1 medium avocado, chopped, plus additional reserved for serving

1 large egg

1 tablespoon Dijon mustard

¼ teaspoon ground cayenne pepper

¼ teaspoon chili powder

⅛ teaspoon salt

⅛ teaspoon freshly ground black pepper

4 whole-wheat buns, for serving

Romaine lettuce, for serving

Tomato slices, for serving

Onion slices, for serving

1. Preheat the oven to 375°F. Line a sheet pan with parchment paper.

2. In a large bowl, flake the tuna. Mix in the avocado, egg, Dijon, cayenne, chili powder, salt, and pepper until well combined. To avoid green burgers, gently mix in avocado. Some chunks should remain.

3. Using a ½ cup measuring cup, scoop the burger mixture to form into a patty. Carefully flatten and place on the prepared sheet pan. Repeat with remaining mixture to form 4 patties.

4. Bake for 10 minutes. Remove the patties from the oven and carefully flip. Return them to the oven to cook for another 10 minutes, until a golden crust forms.

5. Serve on a whole-wheat bun with lettuce, tomato, onion, and more avocado or atop a large salad! Enjoy!

Substitution Tip: Get creative with your bun! A personal favorite option is to serve these burgers between two large bell pepper slices for added crunch and sweetness. You can also serve on roasted sweet potato slices, over salad, or stuffed into a pita pocket.

PER SERVING: CALORIES: 277; TOTAL FAT: 11G; SATURATED FAT: 2G; CARBOHYDRATES: 26G; FIBER: 4G; PROTEIN: 20G; SODIUM: 650MG

LOBSTER COBB SALAD

SERVES
4 to 6

PREP TIME:
15 minutes

COOK TIME:
11 minutes

30 MINUTES

GLUTEN-FREE

GF

HEART HEALTHY

Lobster is a summer classic on the East Coast where I'm from, but I'm always looking for novel ways to use this flavorful shellfish. This hearty salad is a great way to enjoy this sea delicacy when you're in the mood for a crisp bite. To avoid cooking live seafood, use store-bought poached lobster that's been chilled.

FOR THE SALAD

4 large eggs

3 heads romaine lettuce, chopped

1 pint grape tomatoes, quartered

1 large cucumber, cut lengthwise and thinly sliced

2 avocados, chopped

12 ounces cooked and chilled lobster meat

¼ cup crumbled blue cheese

2 tablespoons chopped chives

FOR THE DRESSING

¼ cup red wine vinegar

3 tablespoons extra-virgin olive oil

2 teaspoons dried oregano

¼ teaspoon salt

⅛ teaspoon freshly ground black pepper

1. Bring a medium saucepan filled with water and the eggs to a boil. Once boiling, turn off the heat, cover, and let sit for 10 minutes. Drain the water and immediately rinse the eggs with very cold water to stop the cooking process. Peel the eggs carefully and slice them. Set aside to cool.

2. Distribute the lettuce on a large platter. In rows, arrange the tomatoes, cucumbers, avocado, lobster meat, blue cheese, and sliced eggs. Garnish with chives. Set aside.

TO MAKE THE DRESSING

In a small jar, combine the vinegar, olive oil, oregano, salt, and pepper. Shake to combine. Drizzle the dressing on top of the salad before serving.

Substitution Tip: Lobster is a lean protein source rich in selenium, zinc, and magnesium, but if it's out of season or out of budget, swap in any seafood, such as shrimp or crab, canned tuna or salmon, or a grilled fillet.

PER SERVING: CALORIES: 477; TOTAL FAT: 33G; SATURATED FAT: 7G; CARBOHYDRATES: 22G; FIBER: 9G; PROTEIN: 28G; SODIUM: 670MG

30-MINUTE COCONUT SHRIMP CURRY

SERVES
4

PREP TIME:
10 minutes

COOK TIME:
20 minutes

30 MINUTES

DAIRY-FREE

GLUTEN-FREE

GF

HEART HEALTHY

This quick shrimp curry is a simple weeknight dinner to throw together with tons of flavor and nutrients. Curry powder contains turmeric, which provides a bold yellow color to this dish and has anti-inflammatory benefits. Adjust the amount of curry spice and heat you add to this dish based on your preferences. If you prefer a milder curry, omit the red pepper flakes and jalapeño. Serve over your favorite whole-grain.

1 tablespoon avocado oil

2 cups broccoli florets

1 red bell pepper, chopped

1 cup sliced white mushrooms

1 cup snap peas

½ cup chopped yellow onions

½ cup shredded carrots

1 teaspoon finely minced garlic

2½ teaspoons curry powder

¼ teaspoon salt

¼ teaspoon freshly ground black pepper

¼ teaspoon red pepper flakes

2 cups full-fat coconut milk

1 tablespoon cornstarch or flour

1 pound shrimp, peeled, deveined, tails removed

1 thinly sliced jalapeño, seeded and deveined

2 tablespoons chopped fresh cilantro, for serving

1 cup dry brown rice or quinoa, cooked according to package directions (optional)

1. In a large sauté pan, heat the avocado oil over medium-high heat. Sauté the broccoli, bell pepper, mushrooms, peas, onions, carrots, and garlic for about 3 minutes, stirring frequently, until the vegetables begin to soften. Season with the curry powder, salt, pepper, and red pepper flakes.

2. Add the coconut milk and bring to a boil, then reduce heat to a simmer.

3. Once simmering, transfer ¼ cup of liquid from the pan into a small bowl and mix in the cornstarch until completely dissolved. Add the mixture back into the pan and stir well to thicken the sauce. Continue simmering for 5 minutes.

4. Add the shrimp and jalapeño slices to the pan. Cook for 6 to 8 minutes, until the shrimp are opaque and cooked through.

5. Garnish with cilantro before serving warm over brown rice, if using.

Substitution Tip: Save prep time by using two bags of frozen stir-fry vegetables instead of fresh. Stock up when they're on sale at the supermarket to always have a quick and healthy option available at your fingertips.

PER SERVING: CALORIES: 424; TOTAL FAT: 28G; SATURATED FAT: 22G; CARBOHYDRATES: 21G; FIBER: 5G; PROTEIN: 28G; SODIUM: 331MG

TUNA NIÇOISE SALAD WITH LEMON VINAIGRETTE

SERVES
4

PREP TIME:
15 minutes

COOK TIME:
20 minutes

DAIRY-FREE

GLUTEN-FREE
GF

HEART HEALTHY

Niçoise salads are fun to eat because they're full of variety. From crisp green beans to hearty roasted potatoes, salty olives, and hard-boiled eggs over a lush bed of greens, there's something for everyone. This version gets a quick-and-easy protein boost from canned tuna. You can prepare many components of this salad in advance, including the roasted potatoes, green beans, and hard-boiled eggs, but reserve dressing until right before serving.

FOR THE LEMON VINAIGRETTE

1 teaspoon lemon zest

¼ cup freshly squeezed lemon juice

3 tablespoons extra-virgin olive oil

1 tablespoon Dijon mustard

1 teaspoon honey

FOR THE SALAD

2 cups halved baby gold potatoes

2 cups green beans

½ tablespoon extra-virgin olive oil

½ teaspoon salt

¼ teaspoon freshly ground black pepper

4 large eggs

8 cups mixed greens

1 cup halved grape tomatoes

1 shallot, thinly sliced

½ cup halved pitted Kalamata olives

2 (5-ounce) cans water-packed albacore tuna, drained

¼ cup coarsely chopped fresh parsley

In a small jar or bowl, mix the lemon zest, lemon juice, olive oil, Dijon, and honey until well combined. Set aside.

TO MAKE THE SALAD

1. Preheat the oven to 400°F.

2. In a large bowl, toss the potatoes, green beans, olive oil, salt, and pepper. Transfer to a large sheet pan. Roast for 20 minutes, until the potatoes are crispy on the outside.

3. While the vegetables are roasting, bring a medium saucepan filled with water and the eggs to a boil, then cover and turn off the heat. Let sit for 10 minutes. Drain and rinse with cold water, then peel the eggs.

4. Arrange the mixed greens on a large platter. Scatter the tomatoes, shallot, and olives.

5. Add the potatoes, green beans, and hard-boiled eggs.

6. Flake the tuna on top and garnish with parsley.

7. Drizzle with lemon vinaigrette prior to serving.

Substitution Tip: Niçoise salads traditionally include tuna, but you can swap in another fish for protein. Try sardines, anchovies, canned or grilled salmon, or another grilled fish fillet. To make it plant-based, use chickpeas instead.

PER SERVING: CALORIES: 379; TOTAL FAT: 20G; SATURATED FAT: 4G; CARBOHYDRATES: 28G; FIBER: 7G; PROTEIN: 25G; SODIUM: 889MG

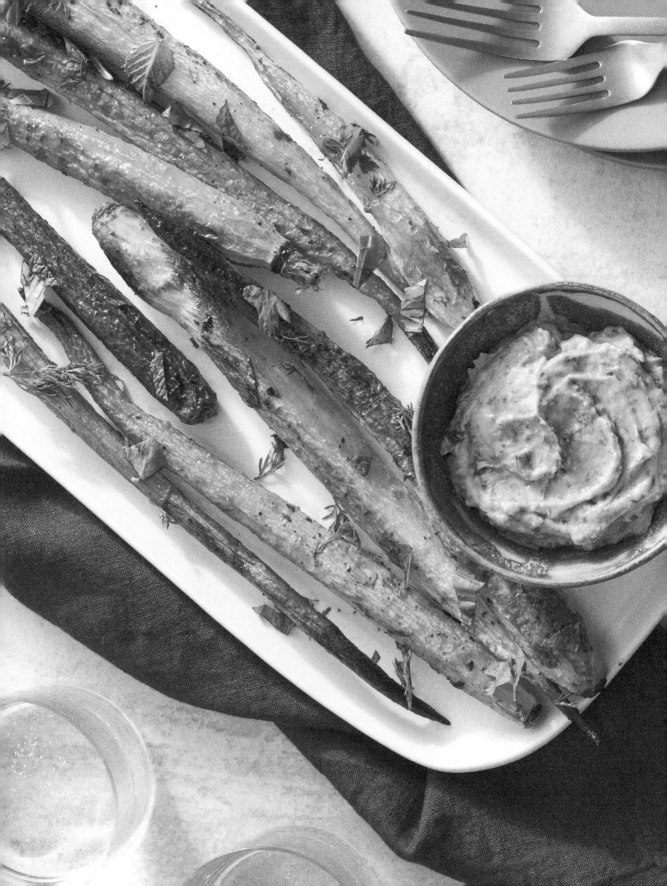

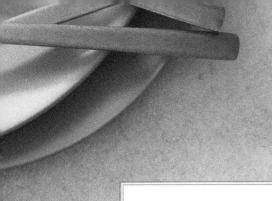

CHAPTER EIGHT

SNACKS AND SIDES

Zesty Crab and Avocado Bites 132

Roasted Red Pepper White Bean Hummus 133

Spicy Popcorn Snack Mix 134

Nut-Free Tuna Waldorf Salad Bites 135

Coconut Brownie Energy Bites 136

Five-Ingredient Portobello Pizzas 137

Whole Roasted Rainbow Carrots with
Avocado-Dill Sauce 138

Easy Roasted Plantains with Cilantro 140

Garlicky Roasted Green Beans with Lemon 141

Old Bay–Spiced Sweet Potato Wedges 142

Crispy Miso-Glazed Brussels Sprouts 143

Simple Ratatouille 144

Raw Zoodle Salad with Avocado Miso Dressing 145

ZESTY CRAB AND AVOCADO BITES

SERVES
4 to 6

PREP TIME:
10 minutes

30 MINUTES

DAIRY-FREE

HEART HEALTHY

Consider these bites an amped-up version of the best guacamole you've ever had! While fresh crabmeat is best, you can use picked-over over lump crabmeat for a quick, lean protein option. Perfect to serve as an appetizer or whip up for a quick snack, these bites will become a new go-to favorite!

2 large avocados, peeled with pit removed

¼ cup finely chopped red onion

Juice from 1 lime

½ teaspoon chili powder

½ teaspoon salt

¼ teaspoon garlic powder

8 ounces lump crabmeat, picked over with shells removed

32 round corn tortilla chips or butter crackers

Chopped fresh cilantro, for garnish

1. In a medium bowl, mash the avocado.

2. Mix in the red onion, lime juice, chili powder, salt, and garlic powder. Mix in the crabmeat until well combined.

3. Top tortilla chips or crackers with the crab avocado mixture and garnish with a cilantro leaf. Enjoy immediately.

Variation Tip: Can't find crab? Swap in canned salmon or tuna instead for an equally tasty bite. You can enjoy leftovers over salad or on a sandwich, too!

PER SERVING: CALORIES: 350; TOTAL FAT: 20G; SATURATED FAT: 3G; CARBOHYDRATES: 28G; FIBER: 8G; PROTEIN: 15G; SODIUM: 570MG

ROASTED RED PEPPER AND WHITE BEAN HUMMUS

Making your own hummus allows you to customize your dip to include more of the flavors you love. This roasted red pepper version uses jarred red peppers to save time, but adds a hint of sweetness. Serve with crudités, whole-wheat pita bread, or your favorite dipping vehicle!

SERVES
6 to 8

PREP TIME:
10 minutes

30 MINUTES

DAIRY-FREE

GLUTEN-FREE
GF

HEART HEALTHY

VEGETARIAN

1 (15-ounce) can low-sodium white cannellini beans, drained and rinsed

2 water-packed roasted red peppers

2 garlic cloves, peeled

2 tablespoons extra-virgin olive oil

1 tablespoon sunflower seed butter or tahini

½ teaspoon sea salt

¼ teaspoon red pepper flakes

Sliced celery, carrots, and jicama, for serving

1. In a food processor, combine the beans, roasted red peppers, garlic, olive oil, sunflower seed butter, salt, and red pepper flakes and pulse until a smooth consistency forms. You may need to pause to scrape down the sides of the container.

2. Transfer the hummus to a bowl and serve with the celery, carrots, and jicama.

Substitution Tip: To mimic more flavor of traditional hummus use chickpeas instead of white beans and tahini instead of sunflower seed butter.

Leftovers Tip: Store leftovers in an airtight container in the refrigerator for up to 3 to 4 days.

PER SERVING: CALORIES: 95; TOTAL FAT: 6G; SATURATED FAT: 1G; CARBOHYDRATES: 8G; FIBER: 3G; PROTEIN: 3G; SODIUM: 231MG

SPICY POPCORN SNACK MIX

SERVES
8

PREP TIME:
5 minutes

COOK TIME:
40 minutes

DAIRY-FREE

VEGETARIAN

Popcorn is one of my all-time favorite snacks because it's a whole grain with 3 grams of fiber per serving, but I often like to kick it up a notch by adding more flavor, protein, and healthy fats. This sweet-and-spicy snack mix adds pumpkin seeds, dry-roasted edamame, and cereal, plus tons of heat. It may take a little bit more time to prepare than a boring bag of microwave popcorn, but it's worth it!

2 tablespoons hot chili sauce
2 tablespoons maple syrup
2 tablespoons extra-virgin olive oil
¼ teaspoon ground cinnamon
¼ teaspoon salt

⅛ teaspoon freshly ground black pepper
6 cups air popped popcorn
½ cup dry-roasted edamame
½ cup pepitas
½ cup whole-grain oat O's cereal (like Cheerios)

1. Preheat the oven to 300°F. Line a sheet pan with parchment paper.

2. In a small bowl, mix together the chili sauce, maple syrup, olive oil, cinnamon, salt, and pepper. Set aside.

3. In a large bowl, combine the popcorn, edamame, pepitas, and cereal and mix well. Drizzle the sauce over the top. Toss together until well coated.

4. Transfer the popcorn mixture to the prepared sheet pan. Bake for 40 minutes, stirring halfway through baking.

5. Remove from the oven and let cool completely before serving.

Leftovers Tip: Store leftovers in an airtight container for up to 1 week. Portion out into individual servings for a quick on-the-go snack.

PER SERVING: CALORIES: 169; TOTAL FAT: 7G; SATURATED FAT: 1G; CARBOHYDRATES: 23G; FIBER: 4G; PROTEIN: 6G; SODIUM: 189MG

NUT-FREE TUNA WALDORF SALAD BITES

Tuna salad is a popular lunch option, but it's packed with lean protein and convenient to prep as a snack, too. This twist on traditional tuna salad is a nut-free Waldorf twist, using sunflower seeds in place of walnuts. Enjoy on cucumber slices as listed in the recipe, or use your favorite whole-grain crackers for a heartier bite.

SERVES
4

PREP TIME:
10 minutes

30 MINUTES

DAIRY-FREE

GLUTEN-FREE

GF

HEART HEALTHY

1 (5-ounce) can water-packed tuna, drained

¼ cup chopped red grapes

¼ cup roasted sunflower seeds

2 tablespoons mayonnaise

1 tablespoon chopped fresh dill

1 tablespoon Dijon mustard

⅛ teaspoon freshly ground black pepper

1 English cucumber, sliced

1. In medium bowl, flake the tuna with a fork. Break up any large pieces.

2. Mix in the grapes, sunflower seeds, mayonnaise, dill, Dijon, and pepper until well combined.

3. Arrange the cucumber slices on a large platter or plate. Place 2 teaspoons of tuna salad on top of each cucumber slice.

Variation Tip: Transform this recipe into a complete meal by loading tuna salad on whole-grain bread or pairing with a salad, like the Shaved Fennel, Corn, and Peach Salad (page 60).

PER SERVING: CALORIES: 114; TOTAL FAT: 7G; SATURATED FAT: 1G; CARBOHYDRATES: 5G; FIBER: 1G; PROTEIN: 9G; SODIUM: 107MG

COCONUT BROWNIE ENERGY BITES

MAKES
10 BALLS
(1 ball =
1 serving)

PREP TIME:
10 minutes

30 MINUTES

DAIRY-FREE

GLUTEN-FREE

GF

HEART HEALTHY

VEGETARIAN

Energy bites are a great make-ahead snack for a quick burst of energy. Made with a blend of nourishing and filling ingredients with no added sugar, thanks to naturally sweet prunes, this version has a chocolatey kick with a hint of coconut, plus plant-based protein from the seeds.

1 cup prunes

¼ cup sunflower seeds

¼ cup unsweetened shredded coconut

2 tablespoons ground flaxseed

2 tablespoons unsweetened cocoa powder

2 tablespoons sunflower seed butter

⅛ teaspoon salt

1. In a food processor, combine the prunes, sunflower seeds, coconut, flaxseed, cocoa powder, sunflower seed butter, and salt. Process until combined. You may need to pause to scrape down the sides of the bowl.

2. Roll into 1-inch balls. Store in the refrigerator for up to one week.

Substitution Tip: Make smart swaps using what you have in your pantry. Use nuts instead of sunflower seeds or peanut or almond butter instead of sunflower seed butter. The flavor profile will be similar.

PER SERVING: CALORIES: 117; TOTAL FAT: 6G; SATURATED FAT: 3G; CARBOHYDRATES: 14G; FIBER: 3G; PROTEIN: 2G; SODIUM: 43MG

FIVE-INGREDIENT PORTOBELLO PIZZAS

Use portobello mushrooms as a pizza crust to enjoy a cheesy, flavorful bite of pizza with a serving of veggies at the same time. Mushrooms are over 90 percent water, so you will have some water accumulate on your sheet pan during the cooking process. Be careful when draining the pan. Get creative and add any toppings you desire!

SERVES
4

PREP TIME:
5 minutes

COOK TIME:
20 minutes

30 MINUTES

GLUTEN-FREE

GF

HEART HEALTHY

VEGETARIAN

8 large portobello mushroom caps

1 cup marinara sauce

8 ounces shredded
  mozzarella cheese

1 teaspoon dried oregano

2 tablespoons fresh basil
  chiffonade

1. Preheat the oven to 400°F.

2. Place mushroom caps gill-side down on a rimmed sheet pan. Roast for 10 minutes, until mushrooms are soft. Water will accumulate on the sheet pan, so carefully remove it from the oven, drain the liquid, and flip the mushroom caps over.

3. Spoon about 2 tablespoons tomato sauce into each mushroom cap. Divide the cheese among the mushroom caps and return them to the oven for another 10 minutes, or until the cheese is fully melted. To brown the top of the cheese, broil for the last 2 minutes.

4. Remove from the oven and sprinkle with oregano and basil. Serve immediately.

Variation Tip: Make mini mushroom pizzas by stuffing button mushrooms with sauce and cheese. Watch the oven and adjust the cooking time down as necessary.

PER SERVING: CALORIES: 221; TOTAL FAT: 11G; SATURATED FAT: 7G; CARBOHYDRATES: 14G; FIBER: 4G; PROTEIN: 19G; SODIUM: 731MG

WHOLE ROASTED RAINBOW CARROTS WITH AVOCADO-DILL SAUCE

SERVES
4

PREP TIME:
20 minutes

COOK TIME:
60 minutes

DAIRY-FREE

GLUTEN-FREE

GF

HEART HEALTHY

VEGETARIAN

Roasting carrots reveals their natural sweetness, making them a delicious side dish or snack. Drizzle the avocado-dill sauce on top to elevate your plate with new layers of flavor, plus a punch of healthy fats. To reduce cooking time by half, slice carrots into sticks instead.

FOR THE ROASTED RAINBOW CARROTS

1 pound rainbow carrots, peeled

1 tablespoon extra-virgin olive oil

⅛ teaspoon salt

⅛ teaspoon freshly ground black pepper

½ cup chopped mixed fresh herbs, such as parsley, dill, chives, basil, and mint

FOR THE AVOCADO-DILL SAUCE

1 medium avocado, peeled

¼ cup fresh dill

¼ cup fresh parsley

2 tablespoons extra-virgin olive oil

1 tablespoon freshly squeezed lemon juice

⅛ teaspoon garlic powder

¼ teaspoon salt

TO MAKE THE ROASTED RAINBOW CARROTS

1. Preheat the oven to 375°F.

2. In a large bowl, toss the carrots in the olive oil, salt, and pepper.

3. Transfer to a large sheet pan. Roast for 1 hour, flipping halfway through cooking.

TO MAKE THE AVOCADO-DILL SAUCE

1. While the carrots are roasting, in a food processor, combine the avocado, dill, parsley, olive oil, lemon juice, garlic powder, and salt. Process until smooth.

2. When the carrots are fork-tender, remove from the oven. When they're cool to handle, toss in herbs. Serve with the avocado dipping sauce.

Leftovers Tip: Double the batch of avocado-dill sauce to use as a dip, salad dressing, or sandwich condiment throughout the week. Store in an airtight container in the refrigerator for up to 5 days for optimal freshness.

PER SERVING: CALORIES: 244; TOTAL FAT: 20G; SATURATED FAT: 4G; CARBOHYDRATES: 16G; FIBER: 7G; PROTEIN: 2G; SODIUM: 306MG

EASY ROASTED PLANTAINS WITH CILANTRO

SERVES
4

PREP TIME:
10 minutes

COOK TIME:
25 to 30 minutes

DAIRY-FREE

GLUTEN-FREE

GF

HEART HEALTHY

VEGETARIAN

Plantains are a higher starch, less sweet version of bananas widely consumed in tropical countries. They're a rich source of fiber, magnesium, vitamins A and C, and potassium. Use plantains as an alternative to potatoes in a side dish, like this simple roasted version.

2 plantains, peeled and sliced into ¼-inch pieces

1 tablespoon olive oil

½ teaspoon salt

⅛ teaspoon freshly ground black pepper

¼ cup roughly chopped cilantro

1. Preheat the oven to 400°F.

2. In a medium bowl, toss the plantains in oil and sprinkle with salt and pepper.

3. Distribute plantains on a large sheet pan. Bake for 25 minutes, flipping once halfway through cooking.

4. Remove from the oven and let cool slightly. Toss with the cilantro before serving.

Substitution Tip: If you're not a fan of cilantro, substitute parsley for a bright garnish.

PER SERVING: CALORIES: 139; TOTAL FAT: 4G; SATURATED FAT: 1G; CARBOHYDRATES: 29G; FIBER: 2G; PROTEIN: 1G; SODIUM: 294MG

GARLICKY ROASTED GREEN BEANS WITH LEMON

Welcome garlicky green beans with a bright burst of lemon as your new go-to side dish that can be made in under 30 minutes! Save even more time by purchasing pretrimmed green beans.

1 teaspoon finely chopped garlic

Juice from ½ lemon

1 tablespoon extra-virgin olive oil

¼ teaspoon sea salt

⅛ teaspoon freshly ground black pepper

12 ounces trimmed green beans

1 lemon

SERVES
4

PREP TIME:
5 minutes

COOK TIME:
20 minutes

30 MINUTES

DAIRY-FREE

GLUTEN-FREE

GF

HEART HEALTHY

VEGETARIAN

1. Preheat the oven to 375°F. Line a sheet pan with parchment paper and set aside.

2. In a large bowl, whisk together the garlic, lemon juice, olive oil, salt, and pepper.

3. Add the green beans and mix together until coated.

4. Transfer the coated green beans to the prepared sheet pan. Bake for 20 minutes, until the green beans are softened, but still retain a bite.

5. Zest the lemon on top of green beans before serving warm.

Substitution Tip: Customize this recipe to what you have available. No green beans? Swap in asparagus. Want a sweeter take? Try orange juice and orange zest instead of lemon.

PER SERVING: CALORIES: 54; TOTAL FAT: 4G; SATURATED FAT: 1G; CARBOHYDRATES: 5G; FIBER: 2G; PROTEIN: 1G; SODIUM: 123MG

OLD BAY-SPICED SWEET POTATO WEDGES

SERVES
4

PREP TIME:
5 minutes

COOK TIME:
35 minutes

DAIRY-FREE

GLUTEN-FREE

GF

HEART HEALTHY

VEGETARIAN

Old Bay is a spice blend made from nearly 20 spices and often paired with seafood, but is also delicious on sweet potatoes. To ensure your fries are crispy, be sure to use enough oil, don't overcrowd your pan, and flip halfway through baking. The end result will be crispy on the outside with a melt-in-your-mouth interior.

1 pound sweet potatoes, cut into ½-inch wedges

1 tablespoon avocado oil

1 teaspoon Old Bay Seasoning

½ teaspoon smoked paprika

1. Preheat the oven to 400°F.

2. In a large bowl, toss the sweet potatoes, avocado oil, Old Bay, and smoked paprika. Spread on a large sheet pan.

3. Roast for 20 minutes. Remove from the oven, flip the potatoes, and return to the oven to roast for another 15 minutes, until crispy on the edges.

Substitution Tip: You can make your own copycat Old Bay Seasoning by combining 1 tablespoon celery salt, ¼ teaspoon paprika, ⅛ teaspoon ground black pepper, and ⅛ teaspoon ground red pepper, plus a small pinch each of cardamom, cinnamon, allspice, and cloves.

Variation Tip: Make these potato wedges in an air fryer! Set the air fryer to 400°F. Toss the potatoes in oil and spices, then place the potatoes in the air-fryer basket, being sure not to overcrowd the basket. Roast for 10 minutes, flip, then roast for another 5 minutes. Cook in batches until all the potatoes are used.

PER SERVING: CALORIES: 129; TOTAL FAT: 4G; SATURATED FAT: 0G; CARBOHYDRATES: 23G; FIBER: 4G; PROTEIN: 2G; SODIUM: 222MG

CRISPY MISO-GLAZED BRUSSELS SPROUTS

These mouthwatering Brussels sprouts are the best you'll ever have! They're tossed in a creamy miso butter and roasted until crispy. While trimming and halving your Brussels sprouts, many leaves will fall off. Don't discard the leaves! Add them to the bowl because they become extra crispy, like sprout chips, when roasted.

2 tablespoons unsalted butter, melted

2 tablespoons white miso paste

1 teaspoon low-sodium soy sauce

1 teaspoon finely chopped garlic

Freshly ground black pepper

1 pound Brussels sprouts, halved

1. Preheat the oven to 400°F. Line a large sheet pan with parchment paper.

2. In a large bowl, mix together the butter, miso, soy sauce, garlic, and pepper until well combined and smooth.

3. Add the Brussels sprouts, including the leaves that fall off while prepping. Toss until the Brussels sprouts are thoroughly coated.

4. Spread the Brussels sprouts on the prepared sheet pan. Be sure not to overcrowd the pan. Roast for 20 to 25 minutes, until the Brussels sprouts are crispy and browned.

Variation Tip: Make these sprouts dairy-free and vegan by using oil instead of butter.

PER SERVING: CALORIES: 116; TOTAL FAT: 7G; SATURATED FAT: 4G; CARBOHYDRATES: 14G; FIBER: 4G; PROTEIN: 6G; SODIUM: 398MG

SERVES
4

PREP TIME:
10 minutes

COOK TIME:
20 to 25 minutes

30 MINUTES

GLUTEN-FREE

GF

HEART HEALTHY

VEGETARIAN

SIMPLE RATATOUILLE

SERVES
4

PREP TIME:
10 minutes

COOK TIME:
20 minutes

30 MINUTES

DAIRY-FREE

GLUTEN-FREE

GF

HEART HEALTHY

VEGETARIAN

Ratatouille is classic flavorful French dish made with tomatoes, eggplant, zucchini, and bell pepper. To develop robust flavor without much time, this simple version uses fire-roasted canned tomatoes, which are just as nutritious as fresh. This recipe can stand alone as a side dish or be enjoyed over pasta or baked fish.

1 tablespoon extra-virgin olive oil

1 large yellow onion, chopped

1 garlic clove, chopped

2 medium zucchini, sliced into rounds

1 small Italian eggplant, chopped

1 red bell pepper, chopped

2 tablespoons Italian seasoning

¼ teaspoon salt

¼ teaspoon freshly ground black pepper

1 (15-ounce) can diced fire-roasted tomatoes, drained

1 tablespoon balsamic vinegar

1 teaspoon brown sugar

Fresh basil, for garnish (optional)

1. In a large sauté pan, warm the olive oil over medium heat. Add the onion and garlic, then sauté for 2 to 3 minutes, until softened and fragrant.

2. Add the zucchini, eggplant, and bell pepper, continuing to sauté over medium-high heat for another 5 minutes, until the vegetables begin to soften. Season with Italian seasoning, salt, and pepper.

3. Add the tomatoes, balsamic vinegar, and brown sugar. Bring to a boil, then reduce to a simmer, constantly stirring, about 10 minutes.

4. Garnish with fresh basil (if using) before serving warm.

Substitution Tip: This dish is flexible to help you use any vegetables you may have in your refrigerator. Try adding mushrooms, carrots, or any wilting greens. If you don't have Italian seasoning, use 2 teaspoons each of dried oregano, dried parsley, and dried basil to make your own.

PER SERVING: CALORIES: 101; TOTAL FAT: 4G; SATURATED FAT: 1G; CARBOHYDRATES: 18G; FIBER: 7G; PROTEIN: 3G; SODIUM: 256MG

RAW ZOODLE SALAD WITH AVOCADO MISO DRESSING

Your next summer barbecue or picnic needs this salad. It's refreshing, delicious, packed with healthy fats, and best of all, fun to eat, thanks to zoodles! Zoodles, or zucchini noodles, are long, thin strands of zucchini that can be made with a spiralizer or vegetable peeler. It's a delicious low-carb twist on pasta salad.

SERVES
4

PREP TIME:
25 minutes

30 MINUTES

DAIRY-FREE

GLUTEN-FREE
GF

HEART HEALTHY

VEGETARIAN

FOR THE DRESSING

1 medium avocado, peeled

1 tablespoon extra-virgin olive oil

1 tablespoon apple cider vinegar

1 tablespoon freshly squeezed lemon juice

1 tablespoon white miso paste

1 tablespoon nutritional yeast

1 teaspoon dried oregano

¼ teaspoon salt

⅛ teaspoon freshly ground black pepper

FOR THE SALAD

2 large zucchinis, spiralized

1 cup fresh corn kernels

½ cup chopped red bell pepper

½ cup thinly sliced red onion

⅓ cup chopped fresh dill

¼ cup chopped fresh cilantro

TO MAKE THE DRESSING

In a high-powered blender or food processor, combine the avocado, olive oil, apple cider vinegar, lemon juice, miso paste, nutritional yeast, oregano, salt, and pepper with ¼ cup of water and blend until smooth.

TO MAKE THE SALAD

In a large bowl, combine the zucchini, corn, bell pepper, red onion, dill, and cilantro. Pour the dressing on top and toss together until all vegetables are evenly coated.

Leftovers Tip: If you have leftover dressing, store it in the refrigerator for up to 3 days. It's also delicious on a sandwich or to dip crudités.

PER SERVING: CALORIES: 135; TOTAL FAT: 5G; SATURATED FAT: 1G; CARBOHYDRATES: 21G; FIBER: 5G; PROTEIN: 7G; SODIUM: 309MG

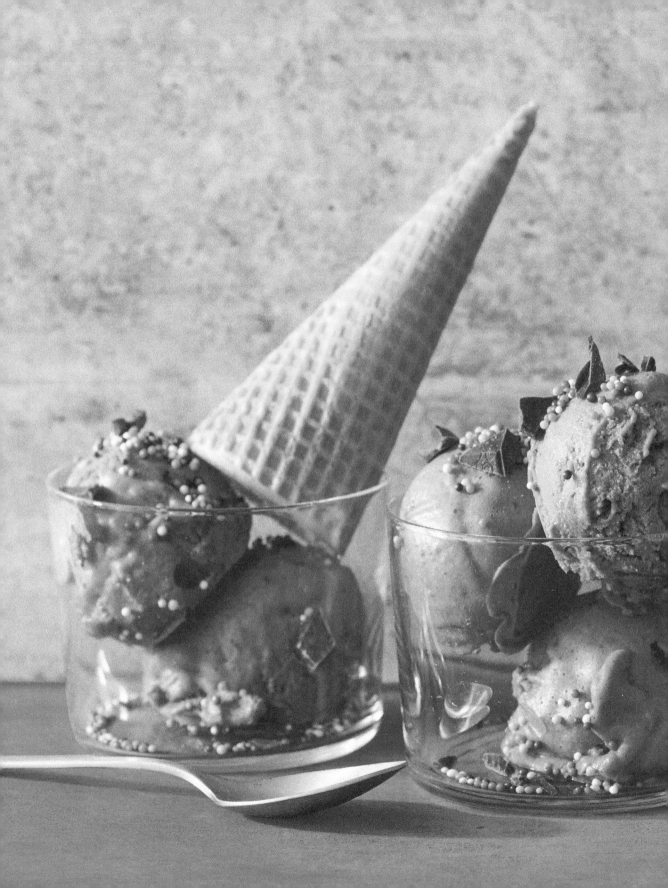

CHAPTER NINE

DESSERTS

INDIVIDUAL BAKED APPLES WITH OATMEAL CRISP TOPPING

SERVES
4

PREP TIME:
10 minutes

COOK TIME:
25 minutes

DAIRY-FREE

GLUTEN-FREE

GF

HEART HEALTHY

VEGETARIAN

These baked apples take me back to fall days apple picking as a little girl. Baking fruit releases its natural sweetness, so minimal added sugar is required for an absolutely delicious dessert! The oatmeal crisp topping jazzes up traditional baked apples so you feel like you're digging into a single-serve apple crisp made just for you . . . with a fiber boost, too!

2 large Honeycrisp, Jonagold, or Granny Smith apples, halved lengthwise

¾ teaspoon ground cinnamon, divided

¼ cup rolled oats

1 tablespoon light brown sugar

⅛ teaspoon sea salt

1½ tablespoons unsalted butter

1. Preheat the oven to 375°F.

2. Using a melon baller or spoon, remove the core from the center of each apple half, creating a small pocket for your filling. Place the apple halves, skin-side down, in a shallow 8-by-8-inch baking dish. Sprinkle the apples with ¼ teaspoon of cinnamon. Set aside.

3. In a small bowl, combine the oats, brown sugar, remaining ½ teaspoon of cinnamon, and salt. Mix together.

4. Add the butter, cutting it into the mixture with a fork. This will get very sticky, but be sure that no dry ingredients are left loose. It will take some time to work in the butter.

5. Carefully spoon the oat mixture into the center of each apple. The topping may spill out over the top.

6. Bake for 25 minutes. Apples should be soft to the touch but not break apart when gently squeezed.

7. Let cool slightly and enjoy immediately!

Variation Tip: These baked apples can even be a part of a balanced breakfast. Pair with yogurt or cottage cheese and add a sprinkle of sunflower seeds or sliced almonds.

PER SERVING: CALORIES: 132; TOTAL FAT: 5G; SATURATED FAT: 3G; CARBOHYDRATES: 23G; FIBER: 4G; PROTEIN: 1G; SODIUM: 44MG

CHOCOLATE CHIP COOKIE BARS

MAKES
24 BARS

PREP TIME:
15 minutes

COOK TIME:
20 to 25
minutes

GLUTEN-FREE

GF

VEGETARIAN

This recipe is naturally gluten-free, thanks to oat flour instead of all-purpose flour. To make oat flour, pulse the rolled oats in a food processor or high-powered blender until a flour-like consistency forms. Two cups of rolled oats will make about 2 cups oat flour.

1 cup (2 sticks) unsalted butter, softened
¾ cup packed brown sugar
½ cup granulated sugar
1 teaspoon vanilla extract

2 large eggs
1¾ cups oat flour
1 teaspoon baking soda
1 teaspoon salt
1 cup chocolate chips

1. Preheat the oven to 375°F. Line a rimmed 11-by-17-inch sheet pan or jelly roll pan with parchment paper and set aside.

2. In a large bowl, using a hand mixer on medium speed, beat the butter until fluffy. Add the brown sugar, granulated sugar, and vanilla, beating until combined.

3. Add the eggs, one at a time, mixing until well incorporated.

4. In a medium bowl, mix together the oat flour, baking soda, and salt.

5. Slowly add the oat flour mixture to the wet ingredients. Mix together on low speed until combined. Do not overmix.

6. Fold in the chocolate chips.

7. Spread the dough onto the prepared sheet pan with a spatula. The dough will spread out when baked, so it does not need to reach the edges of the pan.

8. Bake for 20 to 25 minutes. Let cool completely before cutting.

Leftovers Tip: Freeze leftovers in a freezer-safe container for up to 6 months.

PER SERVING: CALORIES: 168; TOTAL FAT: 10G; SATURATED FAT: 6G; CARBOHYDRATES: 18G; FIBER: 1G; PROTEIN: 2G; SODIUM: 211MG

MOCHA-AVOCADO PUDDING

Creamy avocados are the perfect vehicle to use for a dairy-free pudding. Flavored with cocoa powder, coffee, and a hint of maple syrup, this is a simple yet elegant dessert to enjoy, with the bonus of heart-healthy fats. If serving in the evening, use decaf coffee grounds instead of caffeinated coffee.

2 medium avocados, peeled

¼ cup maple syrup

¼ cup plus 1 tablespoon unsweetened cocoa powder

1 teaspoon freshly ground coffee

Generous pinch salt

1. In a food processor, combine the avocado, maple syrup, cocoa powder, coffee grounds, and salt. Process until smooth. You may need to pause occasionally to scrape down the sides of the container.

2. Transfer to a bowl. Cover and refrigerate for 30 minutes before serving.

Substitution Tip: Any liquid sweetener will work well in this recipe. Try honey, agave syrup, or simple syrup if you don't have maple syrup available.

PER SERVING: CALORIES: 213; TOTAL FAT: 14G; SATURATED FAT: 2G; CARBOHYDRATES: 24G; FIBER: 8G; PROTEIN: 3G; SODIUM: 50MG

SERVES
4

PREP TIME:
5 minutes, plus
30 minutes
refrigeration
time

DAIRY-FREE

GLUTEN-FREE

GF

HEART HEALTHY

VEGETARIAN

PEACH PIE EGG ROLLS

MAKES
12 EGG ROLLS

PREP TIME:
15 minutes

COOK TIME:
20 to 25
minutes

DAIRY-FREE

HEART HEALTHY

VEGETARIAN

Peach pie egg rolls are an easier-to-make hand pie with a delicious fruity filling wrapped in a crisp shell. With a thinner shell than typical hand pies, these fruity egg rolls are a light dessert, perfect for a summer evening! Egg roll wrappers can usually be found in the refrigerated produce section, near the tofu.

3 cups sliced peaches

3 tablespoons light brown sugar, divided

1 tablespoon all-purpose flour

2 teaspoons ground cinnamon, divided

1 teaspoon freshly squeezed lemon juice

⅛ teaspoon salt

1 large egg white

12 egg roll wrappers

Vanilla ice cream, for serving (optional)

1. Preheat the oven to 350°F. Line a large sheet pan with parchment paper and set aside.

2. In a large bowl, toss the peaches, 2 tablespoons of brown sugar, flour, 1 teaspoon of cinnamon, lemon juice, and salt until the peaches are well coated.

3. In a small bowl, whisk the egg white with 1 tablespoon of water to form an egg wash. In a separate small bowl, combine the remaining 1 tablespoon of brown sugar and remaining 1 teaspoon of cinnamon.

4. Place one egg roll wrapper in the shape of a diamond on a flat surface in front of you. Spoon a few slices of peach mixture in the middle of the egg roll wrapper. Brush the edges of the egg roll wrapper with the egg white mixture to help it stick. Fold up the bottom of the egg roll wrapper, then fold the two opposite corners in towards the middle. Roll up the egg roll, like you would roll a burrito. Place it seam-side down on the lined sheet pan. Repeat with the remaining egg roll wrappers and peach filling.

5. Brush the outside of the egg rolls with the egg wash. Then sprinkle the cinnamon-sugar mixture on top.

6. Bake for 20 to 25 minutes, until the exterior is golden brown and crispy. Let cool slightly before serving warm, with vanilla ice cream (if using).

Substitution Tip: When peaches aren't in season, use sliced apples for a fall twist on apple pie. If you can't find egg roll wrappers, substitute phyllo dough instead.

PER SERVING: CALORIES: 121; TOTAL FAT: 1G; SATURATED FAT: 0G; CARBOHYDRATES: 25G; FIBER: 1G; PROTEIN: 4G; SODIUM: 210MG

S'MORES COOKIE SKILLET

SERVES
12

PREP TIME:
15 minutes

COOK TIME:
32 minutes

VEGETARIAN

Enjoy campfire vibes all year long with this indulgent s'mores cookie skillet, featuring a combination of a delicious chocolate chip cookie dotted with marshmallows, chocolate chunks, and graham cracker crumbs. Don't forget to broil the marshmallows on top, but be sure to watch the oven closely to avoid burning them.

1 cup (2 sticks) unsalted butter, at room temperature

¾ cup packed dark brown sugar

¼ cup granulated sugar

2 teaspoons vanilla extract

2 large eggs, at room temperature

4 graham cracker sheets, crushed, divided

2 cups all-purpose flour

1 teaspoon baking soda

½ teaspoon salt

1 cup, plus 1 tablespoon chocolate chunks, divided

1½ cups mini marshmallows, divided

1. Preheat the oven to 325°F.

2. In a large bowl, using a handheld mixer on low to medium speed, cream together the butter, brown sugar, granulated sugar, and vanilla.

3. Add the eggs, one at a time, mixing until well incorporated.

4. Reserve 1 tablespoon of the crushed graham crackers. In a medium bowl, mix together the flour, remaining crushed graham crackers, baking soda, and salt.

5. Using a handheld mixer on low to medium speed, slowly mix the flour mixture into to the wet ingredients.

6. Mix in 1 cup of chocolate chunks and 1 cup of marshmallows.

7. Transfer the cookie dough to a cast iron skillet.

8. Bake for 30 minutes. Carefully remove the cast iron skillet from the oven and sprinkle the remaining marshmallows on top. Switch the broiler to high and return to the oven for 2 minutes until the top is golden brown. Remove from the oven and scatter the remaining 1 tablespoon of chocolate chunks and 1 tablespoon of crushed graham cracker on top. Let cool completely before serving.

Variation Tip: If you don't have an ovenproof skillet, make this recipe in a 9-by-13-inch baking dish. Make this recipe gluten-free by using a gluten-free all-purpose flour mix and gluten-free marshmallows.

PER SERVING: CALORIES: 404; TOTAL FAT: 21G; SATURATED FAT: 12G; CARBOHYDRATES: 53G; FIBER: 2G; PROTEIN: 5G; SODIUM: 383MG

DOUBLE CHOCOLATE-CHUNK
BANANA ICE CREAM

SERVES
4 to 6

PREP TIME:
10 minutes,
plus 2½ hours
to freeze

GLUTEN-FREE

GF

HEART HEALTHY

VEGETARIAN

Look no further for a creamy, chocolatey, and refreshing frozen treat that will satisfy your chocolate cravings . . . with a serving of fruit! Banana ice cream is made from blended frozen bananas. During hot summer months, I suggest always keeping frozen banana slices on hand so you can whip up this sweet treat quickly.

8 medium bananas, sliced

½ cup low-fat milk or nondairy milk alternative

⅓ cup unsweetened cocoa powder

½ teaspoon salt

2 dark chocolate bars, cut into small chunks, divided

Sugar cones, for serving (optional)

Sprinkles, for serving (optional)

Chocolate chips, for serving (optional)

1. Put the banana slices on a parchment paper–lined sheet pan. Freeze for 2 hours.

2. Once frozen, put the banana slices in a food processor or high-powered blender with the milk, cocoa powder, salt, and half of the chocolate chunks. Process until smooth.

3. Transfer the banana "ice cream" into a freezer-safe container, with a lid to prevent freezer burn, and mix in the remaining chocolate chips. Freeze for at least 30 minutes, allowing the mixture to solidify for more ice cream–like consistency.

4. Enjoy in a bowl or cone (if using), with sprinkles or chocolate chips (if using).

Variation Tip: Make this recipe dairy-free by using a nondairy milk alternative, such as coconut milk, soy milk, almond milk, rice milk, or others.

PER SERVING: CALORIES: 344; TOTAL FAT: 9G; SATURATED FAT: 6G; CARBOHYDRATES: 71G; FIBER: 10G; PROTEIN: 7G; SODIUM: 313MG

BLENDER BLACK BEAN BROWNIES

It's hard to believe a dessert made with black beans can be fudgy, gooey, and chocolatey, but these black bean brownies fit the bill! Black beans replace flour for a punch of fiber and protein in a delectable and satisfying dessert. Bring these to your next party and watch the entire plate disappear without anyone knowing there's beans in them!

MAKES
16 SQUARES

PREP TIME:
10 minutes

COOK TIME:
25 to 30
minutes

DAIRY-FREE

GLUTEN-FREE
GF

HEART HEALTHY

VEGETARIAN

1 (15-ounce) can black beans, drained and rinsed

2 large eggs

¼ cup maple syrup

¼ cup melted coconut oil

1 teaspoon vanilla extract

⅓ cup cocoa powder

¼ cup light brown sugar

½ teaspoon baking powder

¼ teaspoon salt

½ cup chocolate chips, plus more if desired

1. Preheat the oven to 350°F. Line an 8-by-8-inch baking dish with parchment paper and set aside.

2. In a high-speed blender or food processor, blend the black beans, eggs, maple syrup, coconut oil, and vanilla together until a smooth consistency forms.

3. Add the cocoa powder, brown sugar, baking powder, and salt. Blend until combined.

4. Mix in the chocolate chips.

5. Pour the batter into the prepared baking dish. Top with additional chocolate chips, if desired.

6. Bake for 25 to 30 minutes, until the edges begin to pull away from the side of the pan. Let cool before cutting into 16 squares.

Leftovers Tip: Leftovers freeze beautifully for up to 3 months when wrapped in plastic wrap and stored in a freezer-safe bag; however, they won't be as gooey when defrosted.

PER SERVING: CALORIES: 176; TOTAL FAT: 6G; SATURATED FAT: 4G; CARBOHYDRATES: 26G; FIBER: 5G; PROTEIN: 7G; SODIUM: 47MG

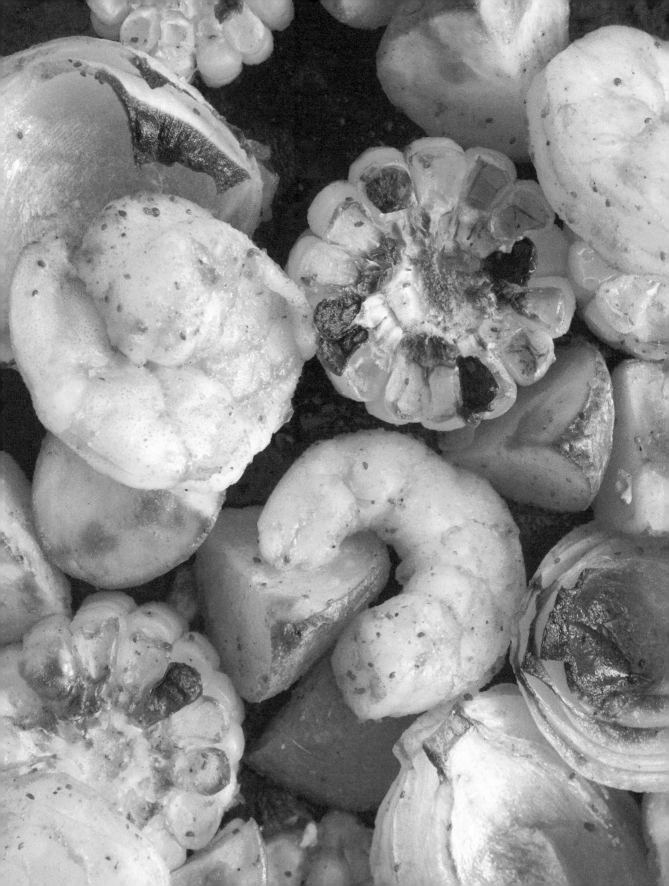

MEASUREMENT CONVERSIONS

VOLUME EQUIVALENTS (LIQUID)

Standard	U.S. Standard (ounces)	Metric (approximate)
2 tablespoons	1 fl. oz.	30 mL
¼ cup	2 fl. oz.	60 mL
½ cup	4 fl. oz.	120 mL
1 cup	8 fl. oz.	240 mL
1½ cups	12 fl. oz.	355 mL
2 cups or 1 pint	16 fl. oz.	475 mL
4 cups or 1 quart	32 fl. oz.	1 L
1 gallon	128 fl. oz.	4 L

OVEN TEMPERATURES

Fahrenheit (F)	Celsius (C) (approximate)
250°	120°
300°	150°
325°	165°
350°	180°
375°	190°
400°	200°
425°	220°
450°	230°

VOLUME EQUIVALENTS (DRY)

Standard	Metric (approximate)
⅛ teaspoon	0.5 mL
¼ teaspoon	1 mL
½ teaspoon	2 mL
¾ teaspoon	4 mL
1 teaspoon	5 mL
1 tablespoon	15 mL
¼ cup	59 mL
⅓ cup	79 mL
½ cup	118 mL
⅔ cup	156 mL
¾ cup	177 mL
1 cup	235 mL
2 cups or 1 pint	475 mL
3 cups	700 mL
4 cups or 1 quart	1 L

WEIGHT EQUIVALENTS

Standard	Metric (approximate)
½ ounce	15 g
1 ounce	30 g
2 ounces	60 g
4 ounces	115 g
8 ounces	225 g
12 ounces	340 g
16 ounces or 1 pound	455 g

RESOURCES

Chelsey Amer Nutrition

An online resource and recipe library with a focus on plant-based, fish-forward, and allergy-friendly recipes.

ChelseyAmerNutrition.com

Monterey Bay Aquarium Seafood Watch

The Monterey Bay Aquarium Seafood Watch is a top-notch guide to sustainable seafood consumption. Search for the seafood you're interested in to see if you're making the best choice.

SeafoodWatch.org

Monterey Bay Aquarium Seafood Watch Sushi Guide

Dining out just got a lot easier thanks to the Sushi Guide from the Monterey Bay Aquarium Seafood Watch. Keep this pocket guide on hand to make environmentally friendly choices when eating sushi.

SeafoodWatch.org/-/m/sfw/pdf/guides/mba-seafoodwatch-sushi-guide.pdf

NOAA Fisheries

NOAA Fisheries is part of the National Oceanic and Atmospheric Administration within the Department of Commerce. They help protect US oceanic habitats and maintain a viable oceanic ecosystem. Visit their website to learn more about protecting marine life, endangered fish species, fishing, and more.

Fisheries.noaa.gov

Oceana Fraud Report

One-fifth of tested seafood worldwide was mislabeled. Seafood fraud is a substantial problem, and Oceana aims to uncover species substitution, improper labeling, and more.

USA.oceana.org/sites/default/files/global_fraud_report_final_low-res.pdf

Seafood Nutrition Partnership

A nonprofit raising awareness about the nutritional benefits of eating seafood. Find science-based information, recipes, and resources on their website.

SeafoodNutrition.org

Sitka Salmon Shares

Quality, wild-caught fish delivered straight to your door from small-boat fishermen in Alaska.

SitkaSalmonShares.com

SizzleFish Seafood Delivery

Eating good quality fish is easier if it's delivered frozen. Sizzlefish has been delivering seafood to restaurants and food service establishments for over 30 years and started home delivery subscriptions to make it easier to eat seafood at home.

SizzleFish.com

REFERENCES

American Heart Association. "Fish and Omega-3 Fatty Acids." Accessed December 12, 2019. heart.org/en/healthy-living/healthy-eating/eat-smart/fats/fish-and-omega-3-fatty-acids.

Burkholder-Cooley, Nasira, Rajaram, Sujatha, Haddad, Ella, Fraser, Gary E., Jaceldo-Siegl, Karen. "Comparison of Polyphenol Intakes According to Distinct Dietary Patterns and Food Sources in the Adventist Health Study-2 Cohort." *British Journal of Nutrition* 115, 12 (June 2016): 2162–2169. doi.org/10.1017/S0007114516001331.

FDA. "Advice About Eating Fish." Accessed October 10, 2019. FDA.gov/food/consumers/advice-about-eating-fish.

Kahleova, Hana, Susan Levin, Neal Barnard. "Cardio-Metabolic Benefits of Plant-Based Diets." *Nutrients*, 9, 8 (August 2017): 848–861. doi.org/10.3390/nu9080848.

Kris-Etherton, Penny M., Harris, William S., Appel, Lawrence, J. "Fish Consumption, Fish Oil, Omega-3 Fatty Acids, and Cardiovascular Disease." *Circulation*, 106 (November 2002): 2747–2757. doi.org/10.1161/01.CIR.0000038493.65177.94.

Mahase, Elisabeth. "Vegetarian and Pescatarian Diets Are Linked to Lower Risk of Ischaemic Heart Disease, Study Finds." *BMJ*, 366 (September 2019). doi.org/10.1136/bmj.l5397.

Morris, Martha C., Denis A. Evans, Julia L. Bienias, Christine C. Tangney, David A. Bennett, Robert S. Wilson, Neelum Aggarwal, Julie Schneider. "Consumption of Fish and n-3 Fatty Acids and Risk of Incident Alzheimer Disease." *Archives of Neurology* 60, 7. (July 2003): 940–946. doi.org/10.1001/archneur.60.7.940.

Olfert, Melissa D. and Rachel A. Wattick. "Vegetarian Diets and the Risk of Diabetes." *Current Diabetes Reports* 18 (November 2018): 101. doi.org/10.1007/s11892-018-1070-9.

Orlich, Michael J., Pramil N. Singh, Joan Sabate, Jing Fan, Lars Sveen, Hannelore Bennett, Synnove F. Kutsen, W. L. Beeson, Karen Jaceldo-Siegl, Terry L. Butler, R. P. Herring, Gary E. Fraser. "Vegetarian Dietary Patterns and the Risk of Colorectal Cancers." *JAMA Internal Medicine*, 175, 5 (May 2015): 767–776.

Orlich, Michael J., Pramil N. Singh, Joan Sabate, Karen Jaceldo-Siegl, Jing Fan, Synnove Knutsen, W. L. Beeson, Gary E. Fraser. "Vegetarian Dietary Patterns and Mortality in Adventist Health Study 2." *JAMA Internal Medicine*, 173, 13 (July 2013): 1230–1238. doi.org/10.1001/jamainternmed.2013.6473.

Pan, An, Sun, Qi, Bernstein, Adam M., Schulze, Matthias B., Manson, JoAnn E., Willett, Walter C., and Hu, Frank B. "Red Meat Consumption and Risk of Type 2 Diabetes: 3 Cohorts of US Adults and an Updated Meta-analysis." *American Journal Clinical Nutrition* 94, 4 (August 2011): 1088–1096. doi.org/10.3945/ajcn.111.018978.

Rimm, Eric B, Lawrence J. Appel, Stephanie E. Chiuve, Luc Djousse, Mary B. Engler, Penny M. Kris-Etherton, Dariush Mozaffarian, David S. Siscovick, Alice H. Lichtenstein. "Seafood Long-Chain n-3 Polyunsaturated Fatty Acids and Cardio-vascular Disease." *Circulation* 138 (May 2018): e35–e47. doi.org/10.1161/CIR.0000000000000574.

INDEX

ACKNOWLEDGMENTS

I am so grateful for the support of my family while writing this book. Thank you to my husband, Scott, for giving me the gift of time to finish this book during a hectic season of life and for being the ultimate (and honest) taste-tester. This book wouldn't have been able to come to fruition without you, my number-one fan! Thank you for encouraging me to pursue new opportunities, to get comfortable being uncomfortable, and for always believing in me, even before I believed in myself.

To my parents, for teaching me the value of hard work and how to cook. Some of my favorite childhood memories are in the kitchen with both of you. Thank you for supporting me in every endeavor; you've always been there to lift me up when times are tough and to celebrate my successes with me.

Thank you to my friends and dietitian colleagues for your encouragement. Your advice is invaluable, and I cannot thank you enough for your support. Collaborating with you is a highlight of my career.

To my editor, Rebecca, thank you for answering countless questions and your support in bringing this book to life. Lastly, thank you to the entire Callisto Media team for working hard on this project and believing in me. I'm so excited to help countless individuals and families adopt the pescatarian lifestyle!

ABOUT THE AUTHOR

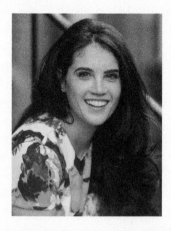 **Chelsey Amer**, MS, RDN, CDN is a registered dietitian nutritionist, avid cook, and food photographer based in New York City. She obtained a bachelor of science in psychology from the University of Michigan in Ann Arbor. Several years later, after personally experiencing the healing power of good food and nutrition, she went on to complete her master's degree in clinical nutrition and dietetic internship at New York University (NYU). Throughout her work with hundreds of patients and clients, Chelsey's mission is to help you feel good through food.

Chelsey started her healthy food blog in 2013 to share easy, nutritious, and food allergy–friendly recipes, without sacrificing flavor. She expanded her business, Chelsey Amer Nutrition, to include nutrition consulting and counseling to help even more individuals. In early 2019, Chelsey released her first e-book, *Thrive in 5*.

When not cooking in the kitchen or working with clients, Chelsey can be found spending time with her husband and son, exploring their backyard of New York City.